¡Cancerlandia!

¡Cancerlandia!

A Memoir

Juan Alvarado Valdivia

UNIVERSITY OF NEW MEXICO PRESS | ALBUQUERQUE

Although this work contains descriptions of people in my life,
many of their names and other identifying characteristics
have been changed to protect their privacy.

Library of Congress Cataloging-in-Publication Data
Alvarado Valdivia, Juan, 1979–
 ¡Cancerlandia! : a memoir / Juan Alvarado Valdivia.
     pages cm
  ISBN 978-0-8263-4189-1 (pbk. : alk. paper) —
  ISBN 978-0-8263-4193-8 (electronic)
  1. Alvarado Valdivia, Juan , 1979– —Health.
  2. Hodgkin's disease—Patients—United States—Biography. I. Title.
RC644.A48 2015
616.99'4460092—dc23
[B]
                              2014047490

Author photo by Joe Felder
Cover designed by Catherine Leonardo
Interior designed by Felicia Cedillos
Composed in Melior LT Std 9.75/13.5
Display font is Kabel LT Std

Para mis papas, Teresa and Juan, and my nurses at 4C.

You live only twice:
Once when you are born
And once when you look death in the face.

—IAN FLEMING, *You Live Only Once*, 1964
(inspired by Matsuo Bashō)

In a certain regard, punk and Buddhism are underpinned by a similar premise: both acknowledge that the planet is brimming with unhappiness. The question is how you confront that misery.

—A. C. THOMPSON, *Buddha with a Mohawk:*
Noah Levine Fuses Eastern Religion and Western Rebellion, 2003

Contents

Part I

Part II

Part III

An Epilogue

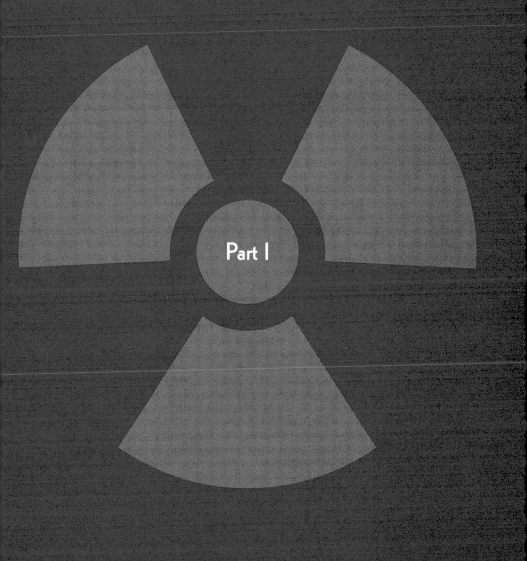

Part I

Three-Oh

THERE I WAS, standing in my kitchen, dressed like a Catholic school-girl—a plaid skirt, white blouse, knee-high socks, cute black slippers—with a beer bottle in hand. My younger sister, Carmen, her boyfriend, Réal, and Brian—who had been my best friend since we were seventeen—were in the kitchen with me. Carmen was dressed like a Catholic schoolgirl, too; she went all out with a red tie, blue sweater, and pigtails. It was early Saturday evening, April 4, 2009. My thirtieth birthday. Since it was a themed party, I encouraged my peeps to come dressed in drag or as Catholic schoolgirls or characters from any Stanley Kubrick film (my favorite film director). I was expecting about fifteen more of my friends and family—including Paola, who I had been dating for less than a month—to show up to the San Francisco flat I shared with my three roommates.

I leaned against the kitchen table, which was teeming with paper plates, chips, sodas, and bottles of alcohol. Brian leaned against the counter opposite me, holding a beer. Carmen and Réal poured themselves drinks while I skipped a song on my iPod.

"I'm wearing my old black bra," I said to Brian. "You remember?"

"Oh, I remember," Brian said, grinning, then taking a sip from his beer.

I cupped and pushed up on my bra to make my breasts more delightfully perky. Carmen shook her head in an "oh-brother" way. The $1.99 lacy black bra I stole from Thrift Town when I was seventeen was stuffed with the dress socks I wore to the community center for which I wrote grants. Back in our zit-faced years, I occasionally rode shotgun in Brian's old blue Mazda while my scrawny, shirtless torso hung out the window. Donning that black bra, I hollered at our classmates in the school parking lot to pass the time. Since then, we had visibly changed. I had filled in my slender, 5'7" frame by gaining thirty post–high school pounds—even gave birth to a minor Buddha paunch. Brian's tall frame had filled in, too, and his light-brown hair was thinning.

"You remember when you used to say you wouldn't live to thirty?" Brian asked.

I shook my head and gave a laugh. I used to say that in my early twenties.

"Yeah, shit," I said. "I am kind of surprised to be here. Now that you mention it, this is kind of surreal."

By the time I was a young adult, I had already had a few brushes with death: the time my best friend, J. C., saved me from drowning at Smyrna Beach in Florida when I was six; the time I almost plummeted to my death—or at least took a ridiculously painful, bone-shattering fall from a dusty plateau in Arequipa, Peru—as I galloped down a plain with my cousins when I was sixteen, my mother and aunt standing on the riverbed six stories below, screaming, "Stop! Stop running! ¡SE VAN A CAER!" before I skidded to a stop at the edge; or the car crash I had in my hometown of Fremont when I was eighteen, my car hydroplaning into the opposite lane of traffic before plowing into the metal barrier along a hillside at forty-five miles per hour. (The dent in that barrier is still visible.)

Back then, I believed I was not meant to exist in this world for very long.

I tipped my beer back and looked around the kitchen at the world I still happened to be a part of. When I looked at Carmen, I could not help but think that the main reason she drove up from Los Angeles, spending time with me during her busy graduate studies, was because we feared I had lymphoma.

I had been having health problems during the ten months leading up to my "big three-oh." First, a swollen lymph node popped up by my left clavicle in June 2008. A chest x-ray and CT scan revealed an "abnormal mass of lymph nodes" between my lungs. Then my left calf became itchy months later and was unresponsive to anti-itch creams. A biopsy of the swollen lymph node in November 2008 yielded a negative response. Three months later, two swollen lymph nodes grew around the area where the previous one was cut out. Then less than a month before my thirtieth birthday, Carmen visited so she could be with me at the hospital for the CT-guided needle aspiration of my right lung—a surgery that yielded a "nondiagnostic" biopsy (which meant that the pathologist could not determine, one way or another, if I had a life-threatening disease in residence). We knew *something* was terribly wrong with my body, but without an official diagnosis, I clung onto any possibility besides cancer; say, a mysterious ailment unknown to man. (*It can happen!*)

Glancing around the kitchen is one of the last things I can remember from my birthday. I drank and drank and blacked out a few hours later.

Before that happened, I remember posing for pictures with my older sister, Mariana, who also dressed up as a Catholic schoolgirl. I remember giggling after I stood with my hands on the kitchen table, head craned back, mouth wide open, and butt sticking out while my sisters snapped pictures of me with a flower pin clipped in my hair. I remember being the only one who drank from the jug of pisco and Sprite I mixed. I remember giving Mariana's husband, Rick, a hard time for bringing "cheap-ass Cuervo," which we did shots of all the same. I remember feeling giddy when my grad school classmate, Barbara, dressed as a witch, presented me with a bouquet of flowers. And I vaguely remember when Paola came into the kitchen with two of her girlfriends in tow. She looked cute in jeans and a huipil, a white blouse with roses embroidered around the neckline. Her curly black hair fell to her shoulders. I remember putting my drink aside and stepping over to her. I threw my arms around her shapely waist and said, "Hi, sweetheart!" before we kissed.

But that's all I remember.

I don't remember hanging out in the kitchen with my friends until most of them left. Or that Paola fetched me a glass of water and led me to my bedroom after a long visit to the bathroom. I don't remember that she managed to get me out of my schoolgirl outfit and into my pj's before I passed out. I don't remember startling awake and yelling nonsensically at her, "You ruined it! You ruined it!" And I certainly don't remember falling asleep with her by my side.

The next morning, with my mouth parched and a slight hangover, Paola and I cuddled. I walked her to the front door where we gave each other a kiss good-bye. I went back to bed. When I awoke during the sunny afternoon, I felt terrible about not remembering what happened the night before. I was afraid I had not been a good host and told my friends good night on their way out. I was afraid they didn't have a good time.

But more than anything, I was worried—uh-oh worried—about what I *may* have done.

I have a history of crazy antics and saying fucked-up shit when I black out. Like running headfirst, full-speed into a garage door after a night out with one of my cousins in Arequipa when I was twenty-two. Or, while on a date, pouring a pint on some guy's back at a bar after he bought it for me, even though I said, "No thanks, I'm too drunk." Or the time I came to from a blackout in an emergency room in Munich with a broken nose and a bruised eye on my first night at Oktoberfest when I was twenty-four. And that's just the beginning. There are *far* worse things I've done while drunk.

I began to piece together my thirtieth birthday with calls I made to Carmen, Brian, and Mariana while I cleaned our kitchen.

Carmen told me that she and Réal had a great time. When I asked if I got out of hand, she told me the only thing I did was toss a plastic cup full of water behind my back in the kitchen when a friend of mine suggested I drink it. It clanged off of a door and didn't splash anyone. She explained that she calmed me down and made me laugh by saying, "Come on, don't be a caca-face."

After I cleaned up the kitchen, I walked to my room. I grabbed the Macy's box on top of my dirty retro lounge chair. Soft-white tissue paper was spilling out of it. I opened it and saw the stylish striped black jacket that I vaguely remembered Paola had given me. When I held it up, I saw an unopened envelope. It read, "For Juanito, from Paola."

She wrote:

Happy birthday, sweet pea!
I hope this turns out to be an awesome year. Another year means more time to enjoy life and the people you care about (like your pumpkin!) :) Take care of yourself and take it easy. You've managed to infiltrate me like the sunlight in my room in the mornings!
Te quiero, Paola

I smiled. I was overcome with joy and a sense of validation (she said she loved me!). I called to thank her for the beautiful card. And to inquire—gulp—about our night together.

"Was I—all right?" I asked. I sat on the hardwood floor with my back against my dresser. I stared at the sunlight streaming through my bedroom window.

"You were really drunk by the time I got there," she said. "But you were very happy to see me, kissing me in front of everyone."

I laughed, relieved that she didn't immediately say anything bad.

"Yeah, Carmen told me the same thing. I kind of remember when you came in. But what happened after that?"

"You pulled me to a corner in the kitchen. You told me you had done some thinking and that you'd be honored to be my boyfriend. We hung out there with your friends until you went to the bathroom for a while."

"Oh yeah, I must have thrown up, because I'm feeling surprisingly okay today," I said, scratching my head. "My friend Andy called me earlier to ask if I was okay. He said I was in there for a while."

"You were. I tried to get you to bed when you got out, but then you started saying that none of this—even our relationship—matters."

I shook my head and stood up to pace about my room.

"Oh god, I'm sorry. I've been told that I get like that when I'm really, really drunk. It's like I have a French existentialist inside of me or something."

I apologized to Paola. Told her I regretted how drunk I got, regretted that I couldn't remember much of my thirtieth birthday party—the only one I had ever thrown for myself. I told her that even though I had turned thirty, it was sobering to know that I still carried some bad habits from my twenties, but I was determined to leave them behind. It would assuredly take some time. This change wouldn't happen like a finger snap, as much as I wished it could.

I believed myself when I said all this, though I had vowed such things before.

In the ten months leading up to my thirtieth birthday, a time in which I had left my job to get an MFA in creative writing—a practice that had given my life a sense of purpose for over ten years—the doctors, surgeons, pathologists, and pulmonologists who attended to me could not identify the cause for my physical symptoms. I appeared to be a healthy, fit dude: I cycled thirty to forty-five miles per week to and from Saint Mary's College in the hills of Moraga, and I could run one and three-quarters miles in fifteen minutes. My body didn't display any "B" symptoms—the more serious symptoms of cancer such as night sweats, fevers, headaches, or a sudden 10 percent loss of body weight—but all the other possibilities to explain my swollen lymph nodes had been ruled out with blood tests.

That's why, although I tried not to think about it while I prepared for my party, I knew there was a decent probability that my thirtieth birthday party could be a last hurrah of sorts.[*]

And it was.

Three weeks later, I got the Bad News.

---

[*] The Evite invitation for my "big three-oh" had a black-and-white still of Major Kong from Kubrick's *Dr. Strangelove*. He flapped his cowboy hat behind his head while he rode the atomic bomb to his death, hooting as if he were riding a rodeo bull. In the weeks leading up to my birthday, I watched the clip a number of times and laughed and laughed and laughed. I should have dressed like him. We were kin.

The Bad News

THE FIRST PERSON I had to tell was my mother. It was April 27, 2009. A sunny Monday. The beginning of a week. She was parked beside the curb in front of San Francisco General Hospital, waiting for the nurse to wheel me out after my surgery. Behind her glasses, my mother's brown eyes were full of worry. Her black hair was a bit scraggly on the sides since it was tied back in a ponytail. I stepped out of the wheel-chair and into my parents' green SUV. My head felt light like cotton candy from the anesthesia and lack of sleep.

"¿Cómo estás?" she asked.

"I'm okay," I said, my voice deflated.

She gasped as she turned the vehicle around the hospital rotunda. "What's wrong?"

I took a breath.

"I have some bad news. I have cancer," I said, looking straight ahead. I couldn't look at her—the woman who carried me into this world—when I said that.

Thankfully, there were no other vehicles around. My mother was able to switch to some form of autopilot and continue to drive through the rotunda and out of the parking lot and not off the curb. I realized after I blurted it out that I should have asked her to pull over first (*ladies and gentlemen, in case of an emergency, you will find emergency exits to . . .*). But I had never been dealt such a card. *Cancer*—certainly a maniacal-looking joker. The first time around, I didn't know how to deal, how to share that with someone else. When put together, those six letters are incendiary. Like having a bomb rolled up in your tongue, ready to be uttered. Unleashed.

9

My mom's eyes teared up, but she kept driving. Then I told her, in what I hoped was a clinical tone, what happened after the mediastinoscopy—the surgical procedure I had just undergone in which they knocked me out and slithered a tube down my throat to provide oxygen so the surgeon could make an incision by my trachea and thread a metal tube with a camera down my windpipe to collect samples from the mass of lymph nodes between my lungs.

"After the surgery, the assistant surgeon came over since she knew I was concerned about the results," I said, looking out the window down Potrero Avenue, which looked more sad and gray than usual. "She told me they'd already tested some of the lymph nodes by the right side of my trachea. Granted, they're not complete results, which they'll have in four to five business days, but she said they're 99 percent sure its Hodgkin's lymphoma." (The assistant surgeon, a thin Asian woman in her early forties, then walked off as though she'd just said, "Excuse me, I need to blow my nose." I didn't cry when she left me alone in that bed in the recovery ward, naked except for the thin hospital gown and blanket over me. I simply nodded, then peered over at the clock on the wall with my droopy eyes to see the exact minute my life changed, which I have forgotten, along with many things from that day.)

Blocks from the hospital on our way to my home, my mom's cell phone rang. The call cut out before she could reach the phone from her purse. She turned onto 24th Street, the busy street on the east side of the Mission District that teemed with taquerias, murals, Latinos, hipsters, bicyclists, and new cafés that reeked of gentrification. She pulled over by a taqueria to retrieve the phone when it rang again.

"Hola mi hijita," my mother said. "Yes, he just got out of surgery. I'm driving right now. Here, you should talk to him."

Mom handed me the phone as she got us back on the road.

Though my throat felt really, really sore from the surgery, I proceeded to tell Carmen what I had begun to tell my mother. That I'd be fine. That she shouldn't cry. That this wasn't going to be the end of me.

"The good news is that Hodgkin's lymphoma is really treatable," I said. "With treatment, I read that the survival rate is just around 90 percent, even for people with stage 3 cancer. The surgeon told me I'm probably at stage 2, which means it has spread to two areas."

"That's good to hear," Carmen said.

"Yeah. And I'm going to personify my disease. I'm going to call him Mr. Hodgkins. And I'm going to beat him. He picked on the wrong man!"

Carmen gave a sniffle-titter.

At that moment, I had not fully conjured Mr. Hodgkins. However, I knew he *had* to be a man, because he was a conquistador. A corporeal invader. Like all the conquistadors in our collective history, he was a wang, not a woman.

My mom parked near my home on Dolores Street. The hilly street was lined with palm trees and picturesque Victorians that I still gawked at after living in the neighborhood for over three years. The sun was up; it was just before midday. A young woman walked down the sidewalk toward me. It felt like I had *CANCER* stamped on my forehead. I felt like I had a dark, putrid cloud contained within me; it made me wonder if people walking past me could sense it.

It felt unreal to walk up the front steps of the Victorian. A few hours before, I had descended those steps, under the curtain of dark, so my mom could drive me to the surgery ward by 6 a.m. Now I was returning home with the knowledge that I had had a killer disease growing inside of me for *months*. Coupled with the fogginess from the anesthesia, that day was shaping up to feel like some sort of numb, quiet nightmare from which I couldn't awaken.

My mom and I arrived at our home in Fremont. I ambled to the bedroom that had been mine since second grade. Over the years, its walls had been covered with posters of Nirvana, the Beatles, Cindy Crawford, a menacing close-up of Alex from *A Clockwork Orange*, and biblical frames like one of Jesus leading a flock of sheep. When I was a boy, I used to lie on my tummy on the carpet with a pencil in hand, a tin can full of crayons and animal books from the library splayed out around me. I drew pictures of gigantic eagles, great white sharks armed with missile launchers, and fearsome dinosaurs for the video games I used to imagine.

I closed my bedroom door to call my girlfriend.

Before we started dating, Paola and I met at cafés near our homes in San Francisco. We read and wrote together; she was also in graduate school for creative writing. She was a journalist for a local business newspaper. (One of my nonfiction classmates at Saint Mary's—a former colleague of Paola's—introduced us.) As we sat together at cafés, we often asked each other's opinion on a line, paragraph, or word in the pieces we wrote.[*] I felt at peace beside her (though that feeling of tranquility was also due to the fact that my being has always felt at home while hunched over a piece of paper, pen in hand, searching for words to create a story, to express my feelings). Paolita was bright, mildly nerdy, easygoing, and a talented writer. After I saw her give a reading at her school, dressed in a burgundy dress and red heels, I couldn't help but be smitten by her. I fell in love with this dream of us being a brainy, driven duo of writers—like a Latino version of Joan Didion and John Gregory Dunne.

I reached Paola at her San Francisco office. She remembers the matter-of-fact tone in which I had spoken while summing up my diagnosis, how seemingly devoid of emotion I was. On the ride over to Fremont, I had already shared the Bad News with Mariana and my dad, who was in Peru—my ancestral homeland—reluctantly handling business over the house he owned in Arequipa. It was emotionally exhausting to have to tell loved ones such distressing news, to chirp, again and again, the survival statistics for Hodgkin's lymphoma patients who receive treatment, to pull the same we're-gonna-get-through-this! cheerleader act with each of them (though I did add a flourish to the Bad News when I told Mariana, "Let's say there is a God, and God told me, 'You have to have cancer, but you can pick which one'; this is the one I would pick," saying God's dialogue with a stern voice). Paola told me she was driving over to the East Bay later in the evening to accept a prize from her Mills College writing department. She could swing by my parents' house afterward to give me a lift back to the city.

After we hung up, I trudged to the bathroom. In the mirror I saw an inch-wide incision at the base of my throat. It was covered by yucky gray gunk that was holding the skin together. The cut by my left clavicle was bigger than I anticipated, too. My t-shirt didn't cover either of them. They looked awful. Frankensteinian. I couldn't hide that something was wrong with me.

Back in my room, I curled up in my bed and slept.

---

[*] Paola was the first person to tell me to change the original first line of this chapter. The opening line used to be: "The first person I had to tell was my mother, fittingly." She told me that "fittingly" deflated the power of the words before it. I disagreed with her at first—which was often the case. But she was usually right about such things.

Hours later, I opened the front door when Paola showed up. Our neighbor and longtime family friend, Heide, was visiting. We had gathered at the kitchen table, catching her up on the day's excitingly morose events. Paola was dressed in her typical sharp workweek fashion: a short-sleeved gray coat, white blouse, gray tweed-patterned skirt, dark leggings, and shiny shoes. My mom grinned before they exchanged a hug and a peck on the cheek. It was the first time they met.

Mom and I gave Paolita an impromptu tour of the house: the living room where Peruvian metal artwork and a big rug with a llama hung, our backyard with my dad's two storage sheds, and the three bedrooms, including my parents', which had a bust of Jesus bleeding from his crown of thorns hanging over their bed.

At one point, after the brisk tour of our home, my mother told Paola, "We will have to pray for him." Being a practicing Catholic and a polite woman, Paola concurred. I grinned and gave a titter. I guess my mom had already figured that my atheist hide wouldn't pray for my own well-being, even when it happened to be the most opportune time in my entire life to do so.* She knew me well. It'd been eleven years since I renounced my Catholic faith and decided I didn't believe in God—and didn't need to. (I consider myself agnostic in theory, because who am I to say with certitude whether God does or doesn't exist.) I wasn't about to become an avid lover of an imaginary being just because a few blood cells in my body had turned heel.

Paola and I said good-bye to my mom, then rode back to the city in her sporty yet modest burgundy Mazda as the sun set over my suburban hometown. (It was a car that perfectly suited her: practical yet hip, but not grotesquely hip.) From time to time, we held hands over the automatic shift. Once we rolled into Daly City, we decided to pull

---

* On my bedroom door, I used to have a piece of paper with three of my favorite quotes, including this one from Zora Neale Hurston:

> If He has a plan of the universe worked out to the smallest detail, it would be folly for me to presume to get down on my knees and attempt to revise it. That, to me, seems the highest form of sacrilege. So I do not pray. I accept the means at my disposal for working out my destiny. It seems to me that I have been given a mind and willpower for that very purpose. I do not expect God to single me out and grant me advantages over my fellow men. Prayer is for those who need it. Prayer seems to me a cry of weakness, and an attempt to avoid, by trickery, the rules of the game as laid down.

13

off the freeway to grab some In-N-Out burgers. "After getting diagnosed with cancer, my ass deserves some comfort food," I said with a smirk. Paola didn't laugh like I hoped she would.

We rode to the flat she shared with three roommates. We went to her room. Bathed in soft light from her Hello Kitty lamp, we cuddled on the bed. While we lay next to each other, I tugged my shirt up to try to conceal the scar at the base of my throat.

"It looks bad, huh?" I asked, looking away from her brown eyes, those big, beautiful eyelashes of hers. Paola peered at the incision.

"It's not that bad."

My lips made a half-frown.

"Now that I have cancer, are you going to leave me?" I asked in a jokey tone.

She smiled and gave me an are-you-kidding look.

I didn't know it then, but earlier that day, Paola went on Facebook and posted a picture of us at the Mint, San Francisco's preeminent karaoke bar. (They pride themselves on being open 365 days a year.) It was a picture taken weeks before: our first "couple picture"—our arms around each other, smiling at the camera.

Before long, midnight approached. I had to decide if I was going to stay over. My home was ten blocks away. This was usually a simple decision, but tonight it felt like a *BIG DEAL*.

Lying on my back, I stared at the white ceiling. *Should I stay or go?* Though I wanted to stay over, it didn't feel right to stay on the day my life was forever changed. Being diagnosed with a killer disease felt so personal; it felt like something I should try to keep to myself. Once I figured I would be on my own—without my family, without my loved ones—throughout the majority of this drawn-out struggle for my life, I convinced myself to leave. But more importantly, I didn't want to burden Paola. On the first night we knew I had lymphoma, I didn't want to set what I thought would be a troublesome precedent on our relationship. I didn't want her to think I would be dependent on her now that we knew my body was going haywire. I needed her to know that I would be strong from the get-go. *I* needed that belief. Like any serious relationship, I had lofty hopes for Paola and myself, even though we were only in our honeymoon phase (though my diagnosis snipped that for us). As much as I could help it, I didn't want my cancer to change our blossoming relationship, let alone destroy it.

"I'm gonna go home," I said, sitting up, grimacing from bending my neck where the doctors had cut into me.

"Are you sure?" she asked, sitting up next to me.

I sighed, bending over to put my shoes on. "Yeah."

"Want me to drop you off?"

"Nah, I'm okay. It's not a long walk. I wouldn't want you to lose your parking spot." (They were difficult to find that late at night in her neighborhood.)

Paola followed as I descended the stairs. We kissed and said good night at the front door. She looked a little sad, watching me turn to walk away as I did my best to look stoic and not somber.

With my backpack slung over my back and my iPod in hand, I walked home down Guerrero Street. The quiet street, lined with Victorians that stood like sentries, was empty. An occasional beam of headlights passed by. I was a lone shadow walking through those pools of yellow-orange streetlight. The first song that came up on shuffle play was "Show" by Beth Gibbons and Rustin Man. It was an uncannily perfect song to match my spirit at that moment—a somber piano, a haunting cello, Gibbon's raspy, worn, defeated voice. It was one of those transcendent moments when a song, written and performed by others, seems to have been created just for you at the precise moment you are listening to it.

The next morning, once my eyes slowly opened, I looked at the soft sunlight falling on my pillow. I lay there, staring vacantly at the light until I remembered that everything that had happened the day before was not a dream.

Let's Talk Death, Specifically Mine

Death is not mysterious. We all understand death far too well and spend chunks of life resisting, ignoring, or explaining away the knowledge.

—KATHERINE DUNN, *GEEK LOVE*, 2002

EVER SINCE I was a teenager, I've always thought it would be righteous to have a bombastic funeral. A celebration, a party—*not* a boo-hoo gathering. I want people to get laid because of my death. I want them to have a damn good time. See, for me, it has always made more sense to remember the dead by laughing and sharing stories about the dumb shit and silly things they did during their stay on Planet Earth instead of being wholly somber about their passing. In honoring the recently deceased, what strikes me as most pertinent is to remember how they touched and enlivened our lives. That seems something to be grateful for instead of sad about, though, of course, there must be a place for sorrow. Pain and suffering are quite the prodigious teachers.

So in this spirit, I've come up with a few things I want for my death. (I am aware that funerals and ceremonies are for the living, not the dead, but allow me to indulge.)

First off, I would like to be cremated. Buying a coffin and paying for a plot of land has always seemed haughty and wasteful to me, though if I were to be buried, I would love to be buried in a mariachi suit—a fine one you can only buy in Guadalajara, Jalisco, the town where I was born, the birthplace of mariachi. I want to be roasted to dust with my stuffed toy monkey, Monito. He was my first toy. I used to sleep with my arm around him in the cradle. He is a somber, dramatico, green-furred ape with teardrops falling from his eyes and his mouth drooped like an eternally sad clown. Long ago, Monito was new, but now he is old and worn from the thrashings I gave him as a depraved, attention-seeking teenager.* By being cremated with him, a neat little circle would come to a close.

Now if I *really* had my way in repose, I would like my ashes to be scattered near the top of the Salkantay Trail in Cusco, Peru. I hiked that trail on my way to Machu Picchu in 2007 (including eight kilometers on a sprained ankle). Though I don't believe in an afterlife, those plains, covered in mist and clouds, surrounded by snow-capped mountains strewn with boulders that feel *alive* to me (my Andean ancestors believed the mountains were our ancestors, alive and watching over us), would be my heaven on earth. I can imagine my spirit happy there, running and bounding through its crisp air, chucking rocks everywhere with a chuño covering my head.

My parents know about these wishes of mine. And they know I'm serious about it.

When I've thought about my death, about the subsequent wake, it's usually been fanciful, though. Typically for kicks. Usually from hearing a song I love like the Rolling Stones's "(I Can't Get No) Satisfaction" or Duke Ellington and His Orchestra playing "East St. Louis Toodle-Oo." It's songs like these that I've often daydreamt about having played at my wake because I feel like they could define me. But sometimes, I have gotten swept up in emotion while listening to a song like the Beatles's "Across the Universe," Rainbow's "Catch the Rainbow," or Chopin's "Raindrop" prelude and thought, damn, this would be a fine song to listen to on my deathbed.

Long before I had lymphoma, I think I considered death a bit more than others because of those fleeting brushes con la muerte earlier in my life. For years, I thought it was instructive and healthy to remember that one day we all will die. I still feel it's a useful reminder.

But being diagnosed with a life-threatening disease at age thirty was something else.

---

* I used to take him to high school during my junior and senior years. Together, we walked the halls, his body dangling from the long arm I held. Between classes, to make my friends laugh, I would bang his plastic head against my locker (I also banged my head on the locker on a number of occasions with the same purpose). I flailed Monito so often that the seams around his neck and wrists came undone. He lost many of the little balls of stuffing in his body. Now he has old rubber bands tied around his neck and wrists to keep any more stuffing from falling out. I have been a terrible father to him. : /

18

Why? (The Inevitable Why)

HODGKIN'S LYMPHOMA. CANCER. *ME? At age thirty?*

After I was diagnosed with stage 2A Hodgkin's lymphoma, a rare disease that annually comprises 1 percent of all cancer diagnoses in the United States, these questions inevitably plagued my mind: Why? How could this happen?

Hodgkin's lymphoma was first described in 1832. And 183 years later, the medical field still has little idea what causes this blood cancer.

Though it was comforting to finally know what was wrong with me, especially since Hodgkin's lymphoma is a very treatable disease, it has always been unsettling to not know *how* it happened—what caused it, so that I could know what to change in my life. Like eat more organic food. Sleep better on a consistent basis. Stop drinking alcohol altogether. Or move out of urban centers.

Even though the medical community doesn't know what causes lymphoma, this didn't deter me from spawning a slew of theories. Could my disease have originated from the cosmetic Teflon plate that was fused with my chest plate when I was fifteen? (I was born with pectus carinatum, colloquially known as "pigeon chest.") Did the electromagnetic radiation emitted from my cell phone somehow react with it in order to create a toxic environment within my chest? Was it because of my lacto-ovo vegetarian diet? The cigarettes I puffed on occasion? Was my body too sensitive to such toxins? Or did my cells go haywire because of the Nalgene plastic bottle I had for years, the one that had strange white flecks floating in the water, the same bottle the company pulled off the shelves in 2008 because of fears that BPA—a chemical used to produce them—caused cancer and increased the risks of other serious health problems? Or was it from all the car exhaust I had inhaled while cycling in the city the prior five years? From deeply inhaling dry-erase markers at the workplace—something I did to make my coworkers laugh? Was it all those years of chewing my fingernails, even my toenails? Or all those boogers I've eaten since I was kid? Or was it all those school lunches I ate in high school? Did someone put a *curse* on me?

How did this happen?

Or was my mother right—that my disease was a "test from God," an opportunity to look up to the sky and acknowledge that He exists? This is what she thought cancer *must* mean—that it was some sort of divine intervention and unspoken communication in the form of a killer disease to awaken a wayward being like me. As if God's mighty hand, His all-powerful index finger, extended through the clouds and pointed down at me. *ZAP! You petty mortal! You who doubt my existence! You shall have lymphoma, a rare form of cancer!* Could there actually be such a sick God—male, female, hermaphrodite, or whatever—who is so greedy, so in need of *my* miniscule attention and belief? Am I "wrong" in my atheistic belief, as my mother said? Part of the losing team? And if there is such an insecure, spiteful God, why would I possibly want to be any part of it?[*]

Or might my disease be a masterful concoction of my own, born from my self-destructive spirit—the "suicide impulse" that Paola recognized early in our relationship? During the time my cells must have first mutated into cancerous ones—months before the first swollen lymph node popped up—I was getting fucked-up, I-don't-remember-how-I-got-home drunk once or twice a week. Sometimes thrice. The troubling part is I often cycled to the bars, which meant my rides back home were through a thick fog of memory. One night, I rode out from North Beach. I must have cycled beneath the towering buildings in the Financial District, down windy Market Street, taken Valencia Street through the Mission—a four-mile ride—without remembering one thing when I awoke in my bed the next morning.

Throughout my young adult life, there have been times—however fleetingly—when I haven't cared about living (which, as writer Asha

---

[*] "And if there were a God, I think it very unlikely that He would have such an uneasy vanity as to be offended by those who doubt His existence."—Bertrand Russell

Bandele pointed out in her memoir *The Prisoner's Wife*, is different from wanting to die). Moments when all the destruction and suffering and injustice I read about, see, and feel from this world is too much. Moments when I have seen little point in continuing to be a part of this evolution, which feels more like a mass extinction.

Could my disease have bloomed from that bleak abyss?

Was the rest of my body too weak to fend off this act?

I still remember a shower I took a few days after I was diagnosed. Pale morning sunlight streamed through the bathroom window while I stepped into the tub. When the warm water hit my bare chest, I coiled in pain. Three red scratches about an inch and a half long ran down my chest. I furrowed my brows while I studied them, then lifted my right hand. My fingernails—since I constantly chewed them—were short. While the shower fogged up, the pale sunlight felt suffused with eeriness.

For a few seconds, I seriously considered if a demon had visited me in my sleep to leave those claw marks. Maybe I had developed lymphoma because someone *had* laid a curse on me? After I shifted my index, middle, and ring fingers into a rake to press onto the scratches, I told myself no; I had evidently dreamt that my disease, Mr. Hodgkins, was perched behind my chest plate. I could feel some tightness, some discomfort there, and I had simply tried to claw him out in my sleep. There are no such things as demons! And who would put a curse on me?

But when I stepped out of the shower to finish drying off, I felt a flash of panic when I looked over at the fogged-up mirror, my smudgy reflection, and thought it reflected a dark figure walking toward me through the fog.

Mr. Hodgkins

*Ladies and gentlemen, in this corner, wearing a black suit, from
Causes Unknown . . . Misterrrrrrrrr Hodgkins!*

SEVERAL YEARS AGO, I read an article about a man who was terminally ill.
His doctors had given him a few months to live. The man was not deterred
by his bad news. He took up alternative medicines, yoga, and meditation.
He also played lots of cheerful Beatles songs and tried to laugh as often as
he could. He spoke to his disease as though it were a living being that could
be reasoned with—a being with its own desires. In this way, he tried to
understand why his disease existed and what it wanted from him. Rather
than establishing an antagonistic relationship with his disease, he tried to
coexist with it. By doing so, the man lived far longer than his doctors anticipated. For some reason—though I never imagined I would ever have to
face my own life-threatening disease—I remembered this article. What resonated with me was the strength he drew from laughter, from having a
relationship with his illness, which his own body had manifested.

In a way, I tried to do the same. Since the day I was diagnosed, I decided
to personify my illness, my angel of death, by calling him Mr. Hodgkins.*

---

* In searching for a title for this book, I discovered that I am not the only one who
has done this with Hodgkin's lymphoma. The first title I considered was "Me and
Mr. Hodgkins," so I Googled it to see if anyone had already used it. That search term
brought up (1) a blog and photo essay on Flickr by Stephen E. Dickter, (2) a blog by
a young woman chronicling her cancer journey, and (3) a blog in a foreign language—
Dutch I believe—that even without the help of Google Translate I was able to deduce
was also one's chronicle of their disease. The telling clues: a picture of a bouquet of
flowers accompanied by gifts; closeup shots of snow on the ground (which I presume
alluded to time's passing—a beginning, then an end); a picture of a shining light at
the end of a tunnel; and then, the giveaway, a photo of the blog's author grinning
while she received chemotherapy intravenously.

The search term "Mr. Hodgkin and I" brought up those same sites along with a page
from gotcancer.org, which sells shirts, hoodies, hats, mugs, and buttons that state, "If
you see Mr. Hodgkin, tell him he can have his !#@$* disease back!" This is unfair

Variations or other names came up shortly after, such as Señor Hodgkins, Fuckface, or hijo de la puta madre if I was feeling angry at him after a couple of drinks. (You will read more on that later, believe me.) I imagined that he originated from the mass of lymph nodes between my lungs, like a sea monster emerging from the deep sea.

One morning, I met my friends Judy and Carlisle at the Red Café, one of our favorite breakfast spots in the Mission. I had shared the Bad News with them a few days before. They wanted to see me as soon as they could. To my delight, they thought it was cute that I had personified my disease. We laughed in our booth while we imagined what Mr. Hodgkins must be like: a well-dressed man, a business type with a white button-down shirt, vest, pressed black suit, and a derby hat. He was like a Blues Brother (but mean), like one of the suits in a Magritte painting (except without a green apple covering his face). I imagined him to be in his mid-fifties, impeccably clean-shaven, and calculating and cunning in a behind-the-scenes-bureaucratic-coup-d'état kind of way rather than a "let's storm the citadel, comrades!" manner. He drank dark coffee in the mornings (dark like his heart!), didn't take off his hat when he read the paper, and was the type who preferred going to the racetrack with a flask of bourbon instead of playing golf. He secretly enjoyed the tabloids just to see pictures of stunning women like Kim Kardashian or Vanessa Hudgens (he liked them young—such fertile blood cells they have). And he was a greedy, greedy motherfucker, voraciously gobbling the blood cells in my body.

I could have attempted my own hippie summit and tried to reach a compromise with Mr. Hodgkins—could've ceded a permanent share of my blood cells, ample territory in my mediastinum, enough space for him to build a discotheque or two for all his other crazy blood cells to party as long as he agreed to stay within his terrain—but I imagined the fucker would have said, "No deal" (although I knew my disease had no conscience, no cosmic purpose, and didn't derive from some supremely fucked higher being who liked to concoct wicked narrative twists for an insignificant being like me).

I was hell-bent on destroying him.

---

because Thomas Hodgkin was simply the first to describe the disease. Another British physician, Samuel Wilks, was the one who did the honorable thing and named the disease after Hodgkin in 1866, crediting him as the first to distinguish the ailment as its own distinct malady.

Ward 86

MAY 13, 2009. My first appointment at Ward 86. The oncology clinic. The place where people with cancer go. (*Welcome to the Cancer Club! Lifetime membership—even if it doesn't kill you!*) In the exam room, I sat up on the examination table, the center of attention. Dr. Attali—the first in a succession of UCSF Fellows who served as my oncologist— stood in front of me. He was in his late thirties, wore glasses, and his dirty-blond hair was slicked to the sides as though his mother had combed it for Sunday school. My mom and dad sat in a cramped corner behind the door while Dr. Attali's medical intern stood beside them. With clipboard in hand, she observed this delicate meeting that must also have been happening at the same time in countless other hospitals around the world.

Dr. Attali made a quick physical examination, which made me feel cutesy in an eight-year-old kind of way since my parents were in the room, just like when they took me to the doctor as a kid. Then he began to ask me all sorts of grown-up questions. He jotted the responses down in my green case file, which already looked a bit thick. He found out that I did not have HIV, drank once or twice a week, recreationally smoked marijuana at about the same clip, and that I'd had three "sexual partners"—as he put it—in the past year (thank god I was already open about such matters with my parents). Whenever he turned to scribble something in my file on the counter behind him, I felt the urge to kick my dangling feet. It all felt so serious yet make-believe. I was pleased, though, that Dr. Attali was my oncologist—the general who would call the shots in this struggle to save my behind. He seemed to know what he was doing. And he was warm in a nerdy-scientist kind of way.

After Dr. Attali completed my medical history, he told us that I would undergo the ABVD chemotherapy regimen. It was the standard for Hodgkin's lymphoma patients. Attali explained that the treatment would be marked by "cycles"—one cycle equaling two chemo sessions. I would have to do a minimum of four cycles (eight infusions), maybe twelve, depending on how big the tumor was. Infusions would be spaced out over two weeks to give my body enough time to recuperate, because each session would further weaken my body, my immune system, and specifically the number of white blood cells—my posse against mean germs and infections. Chemotherapy is a cumulative treatment: once you start it, you've got to keep it going. I couldn't take a week or two off from my scheduled infusions. (Good-bye summer vacation to Guadalajara.) Otherwise, Mr. Hodgkins could regroup and launch a counteroffensive. The doctor explained that I would have to go to the hospital for blood tests a few days before my treatments. These tests would determine if my white blood cell count was high enough to handle chemo. If it wasn't, my infusion would have to be postponed for a few days.

Dr. Attali did not hesitate to tell us that my chemotherapy regimen could make me sterile. Besides that, the main detriment would be the "harsh" effects on my heart and lungs. The ABVD would cause "damage" to both, which is why I would have to take an array of tests to clear me for treatment—and to assess how far Mr. Hodgkins and his deathly tentacles had spread.

To get the green light for chemo (*all systems clear; he can handle the toxins!*), I would have to undergo pulmonary tests to ensure that my lungs were strong enough to hold up. An echocardiogram would have to be done to see how strong my ticker could tick. To determine how successful Mr. Hodgkins's siege had been, I would have to submit to various blood tests (I guess I can't ever donate blood since I'm *flawed, tainted*, not a Darwinian thoroughbred) and do a full-body PET scan—an even more exact CT scan since it can distinguish cancerous cells from normal ones. And I would have to undergo a bone marrow biopsy.

Those three words—bone marrow biopsy—made my parents grimace before I did, only because I sighed and hung my head before I looked up at Attali, pleading *no.*

"Why does that have to be done?" I asked, imagining a huge needle being drilled into one of my bones.

"We need to determine if the lymphoma has spread into your bones."
I nodded.

"The procedure isn't as painful as it is discomforting," Dr. Attali said, observing that my morale needed to be lifted. "What they'll do is stick a needle into your hip to extract a sample, just off your spinal column but safely away to prevent any possible nerve damage."

While I slouched forward, Attali swiveled and pointed at his upper hip.

"It takes about an hour. They'll numb it with a local anesthetic—lidocaine—what they give you at the dentist when they're going to pull a tooth. I'll make sure to tell the doctor who will perform the procedure to wait at least five minutes after administering the anesthetic before he begins. Make sure to ask for morphine to really numb out the pain and discomfort. Otherwise, they won't give it to you."

After he took his time in fielding our questions, Dr. Attali shook our hands and showed us to the hallway. As I walked toward the elevator, a cute brunette in casual business attire that screamed social worker stopped me. She had been waiting in the hall for me—my own cancer paparazzi.

"Hi, are you Juan?" she asked.

"Yes."

"I'm Rachel. I'm your social worker." She grinned, shaking my hand before she greeted my parents.

Rachel shepherded us to a sun-filled room at the end of the hall. The room on the sixth floor of the brick building had a splendid, panoramic view of the Mission District with the Sutro Tower in the distance. It was a beautiful view that filled me with hope.

We gathered in a circle, my mother beside me. Rachel began by asking how I was doing.

"I'm okay," I replied with pep. I felt I was in good hands with her and Dr. Attali, who struck a knowledgeable, empathetic, and—at times—light tone.

"I know this can all be overwhelming," she said, her brown eyes searching mine.

She turned to my parents.

"And how are you doing?"

"Well—this is all difficult to hear," my father said.

I was surprised at his response—the weariness in his voice, in his

27

drooping eyes. I was so absorbed in what I was experiencing that I had forgotten how difficult this meeting—*all this*—must have been for them.

Behind her glasses, my mother's worried eyes looked down at the floor. She whipped her head toward Rachel. Her lips were quivering, her eyes beseeching.

"Is he going to be all right?" she asked before she started crying.

Rachel leaned over and held my mother's hands. I watched them with a clinical distance, as though I were a psychotherapist watching a family drama play out in a group therapy session behind a double-sided mirror. I felt nothing for her. At first I thought, *Oh, Mom, don't be stupid.* I was too detached from them, too absorbed in the moment, in what Rachel was saying, *how* she was saying it, as though everything she was communicating was CRUCIAL. Like I had with Dr. Attali, I was concentrating on anything, *anything* she might say that would help me believe that I would make it. I also concentrated on anything that sounded troublesome so I could mask my worry from my parents with a stoic face. I did have the presence of mind to know that there was *something* wrong, something off in my reaction to my mother's crying. But I couldn't say what.

"It's not going to be easy, but he's going to be all right," Rachel assured her, assured us.

After we spoke about some services available to support us, Rachel gave me her card with the number for the oncology nurse and receptionist scribbled on the back. I felt special having a social worker, as though it certified how fucked up it was to have cancer at my age. She also gave my parents and me booklets from the American Cancer Society—one written for the cancer-stricken and one for the "patient's caregivers." I was also provided with a brochure on the support group that San Francisco General had for cancer patients and "survivors" (a word I would begin to hear everywhere), a handout about getting taxi-cab vouchers for rides to and from the hospital during chemotherapy, information from the Leukemia & Lymphoma Society, a handout about a cancer resource center in the city, and a two-page printout with "frequently asked questions about storing sperm" from the Sperm Bank of California.

Besides the sperm bank handout, I didn't look at any of those documents for weeks.

After we left the clinic, my mother drove us from the hospital to a restaurant.

"Where do I go?" she asked as we approached a stoplight at Potrero.

"Make a left at the light," I said, sitting in the backseat.

Twenty feet from the signal, she began to back up the SUV.

"What are you doing?" I snapped.

"I thought you said turn left at that alley," she said, turning toward someone's driveway.

"No, I said make a left at *that* light," I said, shooting a finger at the signal. I couldn't believe she'd gotten such a simple direction wrong. My mother's lips were pursed together. Her hands gripped the steering wheel, her eyes wide open, full of quiet terror.

When we got to the Red Café, I seethed at our booth—my head bent forward, my eyes glaring off at a spot above my parents' faces. They sat together, opposite me. I was fucking pissed that they had to sit through a meeting scheduled for 9:45 a.m. that didn't start until an hour later and then dragged on and on, well past noon. I was pissed because now I had to rush to make it to school on time. And I was pissed because my stomach was grumbling—and I imagined my parents were hungry, too. I felt like an enormous burden to them. And it was all my fault, although I knew it was not my fault I had gotten lymphoma.

I couldn't say a word to my parents. What could I say to them after such a meeting? (Gee, who wants a drink? HAHAHAHAHAHA-HAHA!) My head felt hot from the screaming I kept inside. I looked away from my parents, from anyone, because my eyes felt like they could sear and implode whatever they focused on. Like the pot of coffee brewing behind the counter. Or the waiter's fucking head if his ass didn't come over to our table soon. We sat there for over a minute, my parents carefully sneaking glances at me, watching me hang my head, waiting for me to say something. Everything felt unreal in a sick and demented way, like a David Lynch film: the warm sunlight that seeped through the windows, falling on the other patrons, on the waitstaff as they whisked from table to table with plates in hand—their smiles, their laughter, their animated chatter. It all felt like a disgusting joke. I felt like something was wrong with every single one of them, as though their happiness was a contagious disease and that *that* was the only reason they were smiling. It all felt like some hideous lie because I didn't know one goddamn thing to smile about.

Then I shook my head and snickered.

"I just can't believe that I would *ever* in my life—let alone when I'm thirty—have to seriously consider if I should freeze my sperm," I said.

I also never thought I would ever have to negotiate a battle against cancer. (*Cancer! Are you fucking shitting me? I'm not even a smoker! I know a number of people who have far more unhealthy lifestyles, and their asses haven't gotten CANCER!*) I wish I could have done it all on my own. I wish I could have spared my parents the anguish my disease had already brought us.

My mom and dad sat quietly, hanging their heads.

They looked like kids getting punished for doing something wrong.

Demons

ON THE AFTERNOON I was diagnosed with lymphoma, riding across the San Mateo Bridge beside the woman who brought me into this world, I thought about what could have caused the self-destructive disease within me. I sat in silence, staring at the highway. I thought back to the months before the first swollen lymph node appeared. A feeling of dread came over me when I remembered all the drinking I had done at that time. *Fuck,* I thought. *FUCK.* And just like that—like a door opening—the most shame-filled moments I had accrued in my life were alive and present. Alcohol was a part of most of those memories. The drunk-driving accident I was responsible for when I was twenty-two—an accident that could have brought serious harm to my two friends and girlfriend who rode with me. The night of my twenty-seventh birthday when I broke the back windshield of my ex-girlfriend Julia's car with a brick because she didn't have sex with me like we had planned weeks before during her birthday, *and* because she waited until my birthday to tell me she was already seeing someone. (Before I shattered her windshield, I got in her face by the stairwell leading up to my flat. Less than an inch from her nose, glaring into her soft brown eyes, I said, "You need to leave. *Now*"—after I had already flung her bicycle out of my home, clanging on the sidewalk six feet from the door.)

Without ruminating on it, my initial verdict was that I had somehow created my disease.

During the time my cells began to mutate into cancerous ones—when a tumor sprouted beside my heart—I was drinking frequently with my coworker Caitlin (a.k.a. the woman who had an affair with me). She

31

was a case manager at the nonprofit we worked at. She was a good-hearted woman stuck in a dissatisfying relationship, just like a number of couples I have met over the years. Our workplace friendship turned into *some* sort of romantic relationship that lasted four months. During that time, we drank hard at bars throughout the city—even ones that were blocks from the apartment she shared with her boyfriend of ten years. Her cheating was difficult to justify throughout our time together; it was the first time we had ever taken part in a covert relationship. (I came back to her, again and again, because I loved her.) And her boyfriend was a decent guy. However, what was most troubling for me were all the drunken bike rides I took once our nights came to a close.

Sometimes this would frighten me—not remembering how I got home. But most of the time I laughed it off, remembering the great time I had with Caitlin. (She made me laugh all the time with her sardonic midwestern humor. And she was a great storyteller. Our relationship never progressed past night-long conversations and drunken make-out sessions in public, though I wanted more for us. Our nights in the city always felt a bit magical when we held hands.) Or I would mentally reprimand myself for being so careless, yet again, with my drinking.

Once I realized that a night out with Caitlin would likely end in heavy drunkenness—five or six pints plus one or two shots or drinks—my twenty-nine-year-old self got just a wee bit smart: I left my bike at home. Instead, I took public transportation and walked to whatever bar we met at. But on occasion, I would still ride my bicycle to our shitface sessions. (The main reason I ride a bicycle is because I don't want to drive a car. I don't want to frequently use a contraption that consumes gasoline—a practice that has devastated our environment and created wars over its attainment.) I was stubborn in my belief that I could control my drinking. And sometimes I did. More often than not, though, I entered that drunken fog, that magical transport machine that whisked me from a bar stool to my bed, along with my then-bicycle, Charlene,[*] to her spot beside the stairwell in our flat.

[*] I've named all of my bikes. It feels like the righteous thing to do, considering the bond I have with them. Like loyal steeds, mis bicis get me safely from place to place, pedal by pedal, along city streets teeming with cars, trucks, and buses that could pummel us with little effort. I feel connected to my bicycles in a way I never have with a car (or "tin cans on wheels," as James Howard Kunstler calls them). They feel like extensions of me: my arms to handlebars, legs to the pedals, my heart, my will powering us forward with the help of the chain and revolving gears.

These rides happened enough times that I couldn't help but ponder *how* I did it. Did I ever fall when I mounted my bike? Was I able to cycle in a mostly straight line? Would I pedal slowly down the street, drooping over the handlebars? Did I stop at every signal? Even notice a stop sign? Would I wait until a traffic light turned green or pedal across when my blurred vision saw no cars coming? Did a car ever come close to hitting me? I presumed I put my helmet on for those rides, along with the front and tail lights since they would be on Charlene the next morning when I would teeter out of my bedroom, but that's all I was certain of. Apparently, I never had a spill or ran into a parked car, because I never awoke the next day with a mysterious bruise or scrape I could not account for.

I am fortunate that I always got home in one piece. I could have awoken from my blackout in an emergency room—an experience I was no stranger to. A broken leg. Fractured skull. Mangled body. Or paralyzed.

I could have gotten myself killed.

When I think about the moments I have been most careless with my life, my trip to Thailand and Cambodia before grad school started, eight months before I was diagnosed, comes to mind. A memory surfaces, one that used to burn with great shame—a secret I had only shared with a handful of close friends. It happened on Ko Pha Ngan, a Thai island notorious for its debaucherous partying.

By the time my feet first sifted through the soft white sand of Haad Rin, one of the island's tropical beaches, the specter of cancer was already whispering in my mind. The first swollen lymph node had popped up by my left clavicle less than two months before. Dr. Chen, my brainy doctor at the time, had run an array of blood tests to rule out any virus or malady as the cause of that swollen lymph node, minus lymphoma. He feared that I had lymphoma. That's why, while I sat

---

Since my testicles are riding on the seat over all those miles—and since I'm heterosexual—I gave my bicycles a feminine name back then. My maroon mountain bike was Rosa. Charlene was a sturdy, gray-black mountain bike. ("Charlene" sounds like a fine name for a strong, voluptuous black woman. Plus, it's a reference from Kubrick's *Full Metal Jacket*, one of my favorite flicks.) Later, I bought a blue Bianchi, which I called Blue, a name I chose because it could be either gender.

cross-legged on my travel towel, gazing out to the tranquil ocean at the most beautiful beach I had ever seen, I had a quandary: *How can I relax and enjoy this when I'm seriously worried about my health?* Everywhere I looked I saw couples wading and frolicking in the twinkling waves, fellow travelers laughing as they ran and splashed after a rubber ball that they skipped along the blue water, people basking on towels all over the beach, their tanned bodies glistening in the sun. I felt like a pretender. An imposter. Their carefree spirit was something that was not churning within me.

After a few days and nights on the island, with its share of morning spliffs, hard boozing, early-morning dance partying on the beach, and even making out with a lady-boy when I was too wasted to tell the difference, I hit up a Half Moon party with Matus and Wyn, two fellow travelers I met on the night ferry to Ko Pha Ngan. Once we passed the gated entrance to the beach rave, the three of us wandered over to a crowd gathered by the lapping waves. A Thai teenager was twirling a thick wooden baton with fiery ends around his shirtless body. With awe, we watched him twirl the baton into fiery circles over his head, along his sides, even under his leg. The crisp ocean air pulsed with electronic dance music. A DJ table overlooked the massive glow-in-the-dark canopy that spanned much of the tiny beach. Rows of alcohol and food vendors lined both ends of the beach. Once we bought a bucket filled with Red Bull and whisky, my friends and I joined the sea of people gyrating beneath the psychedelic canopy.

Drizzle fell through the designs cut into the canopy. Sporting blue Dickies shorts, a white button-down shirt, and cropped hair, my bare feet stepped and twisted over the cool, damp sand. I drank from our communal bucket of alcohol through a straw before I passed it along to Matus or Wyn. We danced and drank in a small circle. This is how we passed the early part of the night until a young Thai woman literally bumped into me.

She danced around our periphery. After our tushes bumped one too many times, I turned to her. The whisky had given me sufficient courage. I smiled—probably shyly—and said hi. She told me her name was Leyomi—at least that was the name I gave her since I couldn't remember with certainty what it was when I walked back to my seaside bungalow at six in the morning. She was beautiful: about my height with straight black hair that fell past her bronzed shoulders. She wore a white summer dress. A large, crater-like scar was visible on her left shoulder. She was a bit young, probably in her early twenties.

We danced and conversed, coming close together to speak into each other's ears over the blaring music. I told her I was visiting from San Francisco. Leyomi told me she was from Bangkok, visiting her cousin. It was her first time on the tropical island. Her English was decent. She spoke with a Thai accent I found alluring. At first, we playfully danced to the thumping, electronic music by twirling away from each other before stepping in to bump our butts together. This made us laugh. Before long, we were getting closer and closer until we began to kiss. I was thrilled by this complete surprise. It is the dream of just about any single traveler to stumble upon a gorgeous local, to ride a shooting star of desire and lust, even romance. (God knows I had fancied such an encounter when I backpacked solo through Western Europe and South America.) My libido happened to be off the charts, up in the mesosphere. It'd been months since I'd been laid, and being at a beach where dick-throbbing hot women sunbathed topless did not help to cool my sexual frustration since every single one of them appeared to be vacationing with their partners, who almost assuredly were getting some ass while the only part of me that was getting any action was my right hand.

Leyomi and I left my friends to buy our own bucket of Red Bull and vodka. I thought it was cute when we drank from our straws—like a couple sharing a banana split. After I got even more wasted, Leyomi asked if I wanted to go to her cousin's house down the road.

It was a small house off the main island road. Leyomi was trying to open a side door while I stood next to a plant with enormous leaves that could envelop a person. Past the house was a shadowy forest of palm trees. While Leyomi fumbled with her set of keys, we heard a woman moaning inside the house. Her cousin, I presumed. Leyomi turned to me with an embarrassed smile. We hee-hee-heed. Then we stepped into a garage.

The light was piercing bright. The garage was practically empty. It had oily spots in the middle of the room and a mattress in the corner. It looked like a place to interrogate people. The only thing missing was a chair to place beneath the light bulb.

Leyomi did not say anything when we walked in. She didn't ask for any money before we made our way to the mattress, where she pulled down my shorts, squatted, and slipped my hard cock into her mouth for a while before she flipped off the light.

The room went dark as tar.

We could not see each other's faces the entire time.

I walked back to the beach party alone. I was determined to find my chums. Though I was hammered, I was not a complete fool. I must have sensed that there was something awry about that romp with Leyomi. After I puked by the waves, away from the dancing revelers, I combed the entire beach party. No sign of my friends. Once I gave up my search, I bought a plate of steaming pad thai and made my way back to the waves. I sat cross-legged on the sand. I ate and watched everyone dance under the psychedelic canopy while a light drizzle fell over us. Then, like Moses parting the Red Sea, Leyomi emerged through the crowd. She had changed into an emerald-green summer dress. She saw me. I set my plate of noodles down on the sand and threw my arms out as if to say, "Well, whaddya know. Come here, you."

Leyomi sat beside me, the waves softly breaking a few feet behind us. I offered to buy her some food, but she wanted a drink instead. Once I finished my pad thai, we stood and walked, hand in hand, to one of the booze stands. I bought her a drink. We immersed ourselves with the crowd and started making out again. With my arms around her, I kissed the scar on her left shoulder and asked, "What happened there?" She must have told me but I can't remember. In time, she asked if I wanted to return to her cousin's. My dick could not resist. I nodded.

Once we strolled past the bouncers at the front gate, Leyomi said, "This time, you have to pay." I didn't hesitate in slurring, "How much?"

She named her price in bahts. I dug into my money belt. I was out of bahts but still had the $20 dollar bill I kept for emergencies. It was far more than she had asked for. I asked if she would accept American money. She nodded. But there was one problem: I used the only two rubbers I had packed during our previous session.

"Do ya have a condom?" I asked as we walked down the dirt road surrounded by dark forest.

"No," she said.

But that didn't stop me.

Hours later, in the middle of the night, I awoke from my drunken stupor. Leyomi lay beside me on the mattress in the pitch-dark garage. Her head rested on my chest, my arm around her. A thin bed sheet covered us. I told her I had to leave. I felt deeply ashamed of what I had done. She told me to stay. She asked how I would get back to Haad Rin, the beach where I was staying. It was several kilometers away. The trucks that taxied people from there were barely running at that time of night. She knew I had no money. It doesn't matter, I said, as I stood and got dressed. I would walk that lone winding coastal road if I had to. Could not give a fuck if a truck barreling around a blind turn in the dark hillside mowed me down.

Leyomi flicked on the blinding light. She handed me the 150 bahts I needed for a ride. I accepted it, thanked her, and said good-bye. I was just another privileged foreigner who had exploited a young poor woman from a developing nation.

I managed to get a ride back to Haad Rin. The early morning sun was beginning to rise above the closed storefronts and hotels, painting the sky in faint swabs of pink. Hanging my head, I trudged along the empty streets until I saw Matus. He was staggering in the middle of a street. He was a young, stocky, good-looking chap. His eyes were half-open, his speech all slurred. He told me he didn't know where we were. I put my arm around his back. Together, we walked home as if I were guiding a frail old man. To my chagrin, I took us on a wrong turn near the touristic center of town. Matus screamed "FUCK!" loud enough to awaken the town. I tried to calm him down with some pats on his back, assuring him I would get us home soon. I dropped him off at his bungalow on the verdant sea cliff where we were lodging.

At my shabby bungalow, I disrobed and raced to the shower. I tilted my penis up to urinate on it, then scrubbed and scrubbed it with soap as I stood beneath the cold water. Mosquitoes hovered all around me, waiting to prey. I covered my face in my hands. My temples felt like they could burst from the anguish and despair I felt, fearing that I may have contracted HIV *on top* of the lymphoma I possibly had. "Oh god, oh god, what have I done? What have I *DONE*?"

The months before that bump popped up by my left clavicle were the most self-destructive of my life. I am certain that all that drinking, lack of good sleep, and coffee drinking I did to function at work weakened my immune system. It left me more vulnerable to illness. I am *certain* of that. Everything else, however (including whether my disease somehow arose from the destructive spirit within me), is conjecture.

But nonetheless, on a mostly unconscious level, the struggle for my life became a final chance to make things right—a final opportunity to overcome the wild, furious, and destructive spirit inside me that has brought guilt and shame and suffering to my loved ones and me in spurts throughout my adult life.

And if I couldn't, I have felt that I do not deserve to live.

First Impressions

THE DAY AFTER my parents and I met Dr. Attali, Paola sent me an e-mail:

Hey sweetheart,

I wanted to talk to you about something, and since I don't think we're going to have much time to talk in private in the next few days, I figured I should e-mail. After I left your house last night, I started thinking that I would strongly encourage you to bank some sperm. I know it might seem weird coming from me, but being in the position I'm in (as your girlfriend), I started thinking that it's an important option to have—and you said you like options. Even if we were to break up, I would imagine that if you ended up with someone else, she would want having children with you to be a possibility. I know you have a lot to consider right now, but I think you're better off taking precautions than having regrets later. I hope you don't feel like I'm imposing by telling you this, and we can talk more later . . .

Te quiero, Paola

I was surprised. It was the first time anyone had encouraged me to freeze my sperm. (*Not* exactly one of those landmarks you want to accrue in life, though.) I took Paola's message as a compliment of sorts, too. As though she was telling me that my genetic seed deserved to remain on Planet Earth.

And I figured she must really like me.

Paola and I would not have much time to talk in private in the following days, because she was graduating that weekend. Her two siblings and her cousin were flying in from Seattle to stay for a few days. Her old-school, traditional Catholic mother was already in town. I had briefly met her the week before over a home-cooked meal of yummy enchiladas.

We said little to each other while we ate in the kitchen at Paola's flat. I think we were both a bit shy around each other, exchanging grins here and there. Paola's mother was a rotund, fair-skinned woman in her late sixties. Her short, thinning, curly hair was dyed a maroonish-brown. She was a widow; her husband had died from a stroke when Paola was in high school. She carried a melancholic disposition—as though life was a form of penance that she had to serve out. Though we said little to each other, she seemed familiar to me. She reminded me of the aunts from my father's conservative family. The side of my family I have never been too comfortable with.

Paola's weekend of graduation festivities began that Friday evening—a warm, summery, beautiful day. Her Mills College creative writing department was holding a night of readings for all their graduating students. Paola and I got dressed up to meet her family at the school. She wore a cute light-green dress and straightened that curly hair of hers that I adored. I wore jeans and a snazzy tan Givenchy shirt, my trusty pair of aviator glasses tucked into the breast pocket. I was a little nervous to meet her family. Like any decent guy (or at least I sought to be one), I wanted them to like me. It had been years since I'd met the family of whomever I was dating. I was a little nervous about being around Paola's mother again.

On a few occasions, I had overheard Paola talk over the phone with her. It was the only time Paola spoke Spanish, though I tried to get us to speak en español from time to time (since my Spanish isn't superb and practice is useful; plus, I find that it's sweeter to say loving phrases in Spanish than in English). With her mother, Paola spoke in an overly syrupy, almost childlike voice. Lots of "Yes, Mom," "I know, Mom," "Just settle down, Mom." Sometimes I could hear her mother's voice booming from the phone speaker with what sounded like gruff, staccato commands. Through it all, Paola—my twenty-eight-year-old girlfriend—seemed to magically turn into a thirteen-year-old child during those conversations. It was always peculiar to witness.

Before the readings, the creative writing department served snacks and refreshments outside one of the auditoriums. Paola introduced me to her sister, Rosa, her brother, Jesús, and her cousin, Cristina. I greeted Paola's mother. Besides small chat like "How was your flight?" and "Gee, it's a really beautiful day," I didn't know where to begin to speak with her family. But I didn't want to come off as aloof—as I can at times—so I took my paper plate teeming with egg rolls, chicken wings, and a big chocolate-chip cookie and took a seat on the concrete border that surrounded the courtyard by Paola's mother. She wore gray slacks and a beautiful, flowery black-and-white shirt. I sat close enough for her to pat my leg and say, "So tell me more about yourself, young man," though she didn't. Historically, moms have loved me. And I've been jokingly brash about it at times, stating it like a maxim among friends and people meeting me for the first time. "Moms love me!" I used to say. And it's true. Or was. All the moms of all the girls I've ever dated thought I was a good boy. (That is, the ones who I met.) The mothers of my childhood best friends thought so, too. (I fooled them!) My record was unblemished then.

Jesús sat beside their mom, but at a distance. He was a tall, stocky, clean-shaven dude who was about my age. A former design engineer at a multinational corporation, Jesús was sharply dressed—a long-sleeve, button-down white shirt tucked into his dark khakis with shiny brown shoes I could have mugged him for. His buzzed head and casual, jokey voice gave him a jock vibe—as if he were the kind of guy who would frequent sports bars on the weekends, make sure your pint glass always brimmed with beer, and maybe tell his bros, "Don't be a fag!" if they ever complained too much about their girlfriends. Meanwhile, his mother seemed borderline giddy compared to the pictures of her hanging in Paola's bedroom. On that sunny evening in Oakland, she faintly smiled when Paola—her baby child—made the rounds and snapped pictures of us.

When we were called into the auditorium, I scurried over to a garbage can in the middle of the courtyard. Rosa and Cristina stood around it, finishing the last morsels of finger food on their plates. Rosa was like a taller, more portly, mid-thirties version of her mom. Her smile, like her soft monotone voice, was typically subdued in person and in pictures. Cristina was warmer, more vibrant and smiley. She had long, straightened brown hair that covered her big gold hoop earrings. Coupled with her trim, fit figure, she kind of looked like one of those stereotypical cinematic urban Latinas who listens to hip-hop all day and chews bubblegum loudly while gabbing on the phone with her girl-friends. I felt relaxed around her, which is probably why I was unafraid to stuff most of the chocolate-chip cookie in my mouth as we hovered around the trash can.

Cristina grinned at me while I hurriedly chewed.

"I can't waste good food," I said, grinning, covering my mouth. They were also rushing to finish their food. After we tossed our empty plates away, I trailed beside them to the line forming outside the auditorium. Cristina chuckled.

"Looks like you're already a part of the family!" she said. This made me smile and exhale.

We sat together in the middle of the tiny auditorium. My hip bone hurt when I bent to sit. Earlier that morning, I had undergone a bone marrow biopsy at San Francisco General.

In the small hospital room, I lay face down, butt-naked on the oper-ating table. My chin rested on my hands. A piece of paper akin to a toilet seat cover blanketed my rear. A small square was cut out of it to expose my right hip to the glaring light above. Once I was settled in, the operating doctor—who had a finely groomed black beard I secretly envied—began to thoroughly explain the procedure, including the tools he would use. Two medical students from Japan stood by his side, observing the procedure. (I felt a bit mischievous about granting them permission to watch, since I have a hairy butt.) He mentioned a four-inch "corkscrew needle," which was *not* a comforting description. In my head, I pictured the screw from a wine-bottle opener.

After the nurse injected a few numbing lidocaine shots into my rear, the doctor told me he was going to push the needle into my hip bone. Dr. Attali was spot-on when he explained that the procedure was more tense than painful, because it was very discomforting to feel something *burrowing* into my hip. It was even more discomforting when I could feel the doctor's arms tremble from pushing the corkscrew needle down into my hip bone.

"Boy, you have some tough bones!" the doctor said. My palms were drenched with sweat. He had to take a break to lower the bed. Once it was lowered, he was able to put enough weight down on the needle to dig into my hip bone. He sounded relieved when he told me that he had tapped into the marrow. I gave a sigh of relief. It was an unusual and nerve-racking sensation to feel something getting *sucked* out of my bone.

Before long, it was Paola's turn to step up to the podium in the auditorium. She read snippets from her thesis—a nonfiction collection of stories about her mother's upbringing in a rural Mexican town. While I watched her read, sitting next to her family, it struck me that they had no idea where I'd been earlier that morning. (To celebrate the conclusion of the biopsy, I asked the doctor if I could see the needle he used. "Are you sure?" he asked. "Yeah," I said with gusto before he showed me a four-inch needle smeared with blood, a vacuous, pink substance contained within the syringe, confident I would never have to undergo that procedure again.)

It was my little secret.

And it felt very strange.

Sunday morning, Paola, Rosa, Jesús, and I waded out in the chilly waves at Seacliff Beach, an hour-and-a-half drive south of San Francisco. A thin veil of fog enveloped the coast. A few other kids and families swam in the ocean. I clutched my bodyboard against my right side as I high-stepped through the lapping waves toward a big one cresting in the near distance. As the wave broke, I laid out on my board to ride it to shore, hooting and hee-hee-heeeeeing along the way. After I caught a few righteous waves, I offered my board to Paola and her siblings. They all kindly said, "No thanks." It'd been years since I had gone bodyboarding. I knew it would make me feel enormously free and happy to ride the ocean's waves. My lymphoma was already affecting my decision-making. Making me different from the people around me. It made me understand how precious the present was. With a trying summer of chemotherapy looming, I knew I needed all the joy and play I could seize that day.

Once we had enough of the cold ocean, we trudged over to Paola's mother, Cristina, and another cousin who sat beneath striped umbrellas. Their mother sat like a matron in her lawn chair. For lunch, we gobbled sandwiches and chowed on some chips. Jesús, then Cristina, lay out on their towels, covering their eyes from the sun to sleep. I was taken aback. Lying beside them to sleep felt intimate, something I would only do with my cousins or close friends. We were tired from all the partying we'd done the night before, drinking and dancing at clubs in the Mission after Paola's graduation. Being with her family seemed so easy then; it was as if each person was an individual piece of a puzzle that I could fit into.

Paola and I rode back to San Francisco in her car once the sun began its descent. We rode along the coastal highway. Much of the coast was veiled in a picturesque, seemingly mystic fog. I remember staring out toward the ocean on her left, past the lush fields enveloped in fog. Her iPod filled the car with songs in Spanish—pop-rock songs about love, rancheras she grew up listening to. We also listened to my copy of Lhasa de Sela's debut album. Her godly voice made me tear up sometimes, because it was so hauntingly beautiful. (Half a year later, she would die at the age of thirty-seven from breast cancer.) Paola really dug her. She asked if she could borrow the CD, which pleased me since she didn't connect with much of the music I listened to.

I felt so at peace beside Paola on that ride. As long as the music was good and the scenery was tranquil, I could have ridden beside her until the car ran out of gas. By then, we had been together for about two months. She had already become the truest of companions—a partner in a way that none of my other girlfriends had ever been. She had come into my life at a time when I needed her, though it was something I wouldn't admit for many months. That day, I began to truly believe that our union was something that was simply meant to happen. Not quite in the sense of destiny—a concept I staunchly do not wish to believe in—but like a natural, undeniable bond, a profound companionship that would inevitably flower if Paola and I ever met and opened our hearts, like seeds in sunlight, to each other.

Now that I think about it, it was also the first time I began to take her for granted. As if she would always be by my side, no matter what I did, no matter what happened between us.

Numb

PAOLA'S HEAD WAS nestled against my chest, her arm draped over my heart, the tumor blooming beside it. My arm was snug beneath her as we lay on her bed. The afternoon sun shone through the window blinds. I stared at the ceiling, remembering how emotionless, how distant I felt when my mom cried in front of my social worker.

"I'm worried that I'm not allowing myself to feel pity, to feel sorry for myself," I said. "I feel like I just need a good cry, but I can't make it come out."

Paola made a soft murmur. She rubbed my shoulder.

Once I knew I had lymphoma, one of the last things I wanted was to feel like a victim. I treated self-pity as though it were something to be allergic to. But even then, lying in bed with Paolita, I was becoming aware that this tactic was going to have its drawbacks. It was as though some part of me had been shut off—the part that could grieve for this world, the part that could feel sorrow, let alone for me. Something inside me was gone. Missing. Vacant.

To Freeze or Not to Freeze Thy Love Spunk

TAGI AND I sat side by side at Dalva, shooting the breeze over happy-hour beers. Red candleholders flickered along the bar counter. The sun's fading light streamed through the door. She was dressed beautifully as usual: black linen pants, medium-sized heels, and a simple yet elegant floral blouse. Coupled with her brown skin and black hair that ran past her shoulders, her outfit effused a casual businesswoman-from-the-tropics aura. Over the years, Tagi (a.k.a. Terrible T or Terrific T)—who is six years older than I am—was one of my dearest friends and a favored drinking buddy. She's one of the few passionate, delightfully crazy, über-intelligent persons who seemed to see this insane world like I did.

I was catching her up on my pending battle with Mr. Hodgkins, telling her about the "weigh-in" activities I had to do before I could step into the ring with his blood-cell-lusting ass. When she asked about chemotherapy, I explained the potentially harmful side effects, such as firing blanks in the procreative department, like one of those pistols that shoots out a flag that says "Bang."

"It's funny, but when I was a kid, going to SF State, I thought about becoming a sperm donor since they had ads in their student newspaper," I said. "It seemed like easy money—getting paid to shoot my load. Shit, sign me up. I'm already *doing that*! And now I have to seriously think about freezing my sperm because I might become impotent."

I smirked and shook my head. Tagi sighed before we tipped our pints back. Then I started laughing.

"We should hold a fundraiser to raise funds to freeze my love spunk!"

Tagi laughed, her eyes widening.

"Yes, yes! I'd be more than happy to make some lemonade to raise money toward freezing your love spunk!"

We laughed at the idea of setting up a lemonade stand with a sign written in crayon that would read something like:

LEMONADE—$1

Proceeds will be used to help freeze my sperm

"I could sell stories or even poems that people could give to their lovers."

"Or we could set up a kissing booth?" Tagi suggested with a mischievous grin.

"Oooh! That's a great idea. I'd just have to tell them not to worry—my cancer isn't contagious!"

We roared.

Later that evening, I went on Facebook and asked my friends to donate to my fundraising campaign: Let's Freeze Juan's Jizz! It got a handful of likes.

As far as freezing sperm, I figured it wouldn't cost more than $300–400 for wangs like me. All I had to do was shoot my load in a container. The sperm bank would just have to freeze and store my "ejaculate." ("Bank"? Would my jizz collect interest over time?) That wasn't difficult!—nothing like Luke Skywalker shooting those proton torpedoes into the Death Star's narrow exhaust port at the end of *Star Wars*.

How costly could it be?

I already had one pledged donor: my parents. After our meeting with Dr. Attali, my dad told me that he and my mom would help cover the cost of storing my sperm. But that's all he said—no rousing emotional speech about doing what we can to assure that I bring grandkids into their lives. No stirring words about continuing the Alvarado bloodline. He assured me that they would help financially, but that was all he said about it. It was almost disappointing, though it was one fewer problem for me.

Nevertheless, I was surprised that Paola was the one person in my lymphoma-tinged world who really, truly encouraged me to consider sperm storage. I expected that from my parents—especially my mom. In recent years, she bugged Carmen on occasion about kids and marriage. She'd ask when she would have grandchildren to care for. My mom pulled that guilt shit on me once after I took her out for dinner on Valentine's Day in 2008. We were at home, sitting on the couch, watching TV when she said, "You know, your father's not getting any younger—and I know he'd like to have some grandchildren around the house."

I rolled my eyes and broke into a grin. "Oh god, Mom," I said, "I can't believe you're pulling this!" And she never brought it up again.

Back then, the question of having kids was one of my furthest concerns.

But once my body turned against itself, I had to confront that question.

Frozen Sperm Addendum

WHEN I THINK about the future, the world my hypothetical children would inhabit, I recall an article I read in the *San Francisco Chronicle* in 2003 when I was twenty-four. It concerned a leaked report that the U.S. Department of Defense had commissioned from Global Business Network (GBN), a San Francisco–based consulting group that specializes in scenario planning. The report was titled, "Imagining the Unthinkable: An Abrupt Climate Change Scenario and Its Implications for United States National Security."

In that twenty-two-page report, GBN's authors relied on scientific research from leading climate scientists to posit a future scenario in which global warming would abruptly and drastically alter the world's climate. Within decades, their scenario projected food shortages and a sharp decrease in the availability and quality of fresh water in key crop-growing regions of the world, such as California. This, in turn, could lead to regional wars over natural resources—namely water. New political alliances would be formed regardless of religious differences or political ideologies. These regions could spiral into anarchy, with groups fighting simply to live. I'm familiar with the report and the scientific evidence used to inform it because I researched its sources to write an article about it. (I needed a writing sample for the graduate journalism schools I applied to that year.) I also researched them to become informed.

Although the report's authors cautioned that it was *just* a possible worst-case scenario (an educated guess, not a firm projection), it has helped to color my world in the way a bible does for a devout believer. In the past eleven years, reports from international panels on climate change have provided little reason to be optimistic about life on Planet Earth this coming century. Ever since I read about GBN's report, I feel uneasy when I'm in the kitchen and someone is blasting water from the faucet and not using it to rinse the dishes. Seeing such waste of water tends to make my eyes go buggy, all while I try to contain a "WHAT ARE YOU DOING?" from bursting out of my mouth. Since I researched the studies that informed the report's findings, my faith in our race's continued existence has waned.

How long will humanity last?

Is self-destruction the most defining trait of our species?

Will I be around to witness our collective end?

The report alone did not accomplish this, but reading all those bleak climate projections was like a gigantic glacial slab of my hope for a better world breaking off into the depths of a dark ocean. My faith in humanity only further erodes when I read or hear the lies our top-ranking politicians spew on a regular basis. Like the lies that led the United States into an illegal occupation of Iraq, lies that killed and maimed and ruined thousands and thousands of lives. Or when General Colin Powell, during the Persian Gulf War, was asked how many Iraqis were killed and responded, "Frankly, that's a number that doesn't interest me very much." Or when I read books that detail the calculated slaughter and torture of New World natives by greedy, power-lusting Europeans. Or when I saw an undercover video of a fur trader in China beating a raccoon dog unconscious by swinging it from its tail and bashing its skull against the sidewalk, THUMP, THUMP, THUMP, then hanging it by its feet from a pole in order to skin it alive with a long knife; once the raccoon dog's fur was wrenched off, the carcass was tossed onto a mound of trash, where it slumped dead to the side, all bloody flesh and muscle. That man tossed away this beautiful creature, this life, like the trash I have seen Latinos and other Mission District residents discard on our sidewalks, as if they're saying, "I don't give a fuck about our world."

These are just a few examples. I could go on and on and on.

Perhaps that's partly why I cry when I am awestruck by a glorious song like the Beatles' "Because" or John Coltrane's "My Favorite Things." Or when I watch a masterful film like Guillermo del Toro's *Pan's Labyrinth*. Sometimes I have felt my eyes well up when I've seen something adorable like an Elmo, Big Bird, or Cookie Monster baby doll—each brimming with radiant innocence. I am constantly reminded that our species is capable of creating such beauty, but I also see, read about, and feel our destruction of life, our planet, and our heinous disregard for other living beings. Bit by bit, my hope that we can better love one another, that we can live more wisely together, has all but dissipated.

That's why, for years, I've hesitated to say that I want to bring a child into our world. *This world. This time.* My god. I'm not sure if I could live with myself if I were to see mi hijo o hijita suffer the cruelties of a world controlled by insatiably greedy men who have made a peerless god of profit and commerce over life itself. How can I bring a child—a miniature version of myself and the woman I love—into a world where he or she could witness genocide firsthand, where he or she could see mass graves filled with charred bodies? How can I bring a child into a world where he or she might someday have a gun put to their head by a soldier demanding water or food? That's where I think we're headed. Our world, with its over seven billion humans and subsequently depleting natural resources, *is* getting crazier and crazier. And what's going to happen when water insecurity sets in at a global level? (In 1995, then vice president of the World Bank Ismail Serageldin said, "The wars of the next century will be fought over water.")

I do believe civilization is a rotting carcass.

I am afraid that I will witness horrific human acts in my lifetime— ones *I* might commit.[*]

And I'm not sure if I can bear to see my children suffer that as well.

---

[*] "You see, Mr. Gittes, most people never have to face the fact that at the right time, and the right place, they're capable of *anything*."—Noah Cross, played by John Huston in Robert Towne's *Chinatown*.

Ceremony

I TOOK A seat near the back rows of McKeon Pavilion among all the families dressed up for the graduation ceremony. The Saint Mary's gymnasium was small but not packed to capacity that Sunday afternoon. The gym floor was covered with gray butcher paper and rows and rows of white folding chairs facing the stage, waiting to be filled by the students we had come to see. Shimmering maroon and blue curtains hung on the wall behind the stage, and floral arrangements adorned it. Throughout the crowd, an occasional balloon floated in the air, like a shiny one that read, "Congratulations, Graduate!"

There was an expectant, infectiously festive buzz in the gym, and smiles abounded. I set my pea coat aside and read George Saunders's *CivilWarLand in Bad Decline.* Or tried to. It was impossible not to feel excited for my nonfiction classmates who were graduating, even though I was sad they would not be back next year.

Soon after, a soft, lilting classical melody began to play through the speakers. A reverent hush came over the crowd. All eyes turned to the graduates as they marched in, all capped and gowned, with shiny shoes and high heels. The gym lit up with camera flashes. I grinned as I watched my classmates look around the crowd for their loved ones once they stood in front of their chairs. I could feel myself get a little emotional as the music continued to play and our robed professors marched between the rows of graduates on their way to the stage. The simple beauty of that ceremony, that ritual to mark a culmination, stirred me.

That was when I realized that there was nothing I wanted more than to stand on that gymnasium floor a year from that date, my mom, my dad, Paola, my sisters and loved ones cheering and waving to me from the stands.

Nothing.

The Dread (of Chemo)

IF CANCER FELT like movie house–sized lettering coming at me from every direction when I was first diagnosed . . .

CANCER   CANCER

                          CANCER   CANCER

           CANCER

                                CANCER

CANCER

                CANCER

                               CANCER

CANCER

                 CANCER   CANCER

then chemo felt like I would be pushed into the foulest Porta Potty, its walls caked with chunky, yellow-pink vomit, my face shoved into a urine-splattered toilet seat, the fumes from the mound of shit sordid enough to make my hair fall out on the spot and make me shiver and retch in a fantastically grandiose way that only Regan from *The Exorcist* could top.

I went alone to my second oncology appointment on May 27. (I didn't want to put my parents through another one.) From my perch on the examination table, I asked Dr. Attali about the percentages of going sterile from chemotherapy.

"I don't know the numbers off the top of my head, but it's one of those side effects that affects a minority of patients, probably around five percent, so it's small," he said.[*] "But we have to mention it because for some people that's a really important decision in their lives—having their own children."

Dr. Attali went on to tell me that he was frustrated that my PET scan had not been scheduled yet. The longer it took to schedule, the longer we would have to wait to begin treatment. We needed to determine how big the tumor was in order to figure out my treatment plan, which could include radiation if the tumor was large enough. Worse, he told me I would have to do the bone marrow biopsy *again*. Somehow, the operating doctor had not gotten a sufficient marrow sample. I hung and shook my head.

But that's not what almost drove me to tears. When we were wrapping up our meeting, Dr. Attali again asked me what I did for a living.

"Right now, I'm working part time as a grant writer," I said. "I was hoping to find some more work over the summer while I'm not in school, but I guess that's out of the question now."

"You're a full-time student? And how many hours do you work?"

"I work fifteen hours a week. It's really flexible. I get to make my own schedule. And yeah, I was going to school full time."

"Well, depending on how sick you get, you'll probably be able to keep working. But school—you might as well begin to accept that you probably won't be able to go back next semester. You might have to take a year off. Cancer changes your entire life. Right now, your health has to be your top priority. It's like a full-time job. Besides, when you go back to grad school, you want to do it right. You don't want to give it half of your effort."

Right then and there, I felt like dropping to my knees and burying my face in my hands. It had been seven years since I had been a student, studying cinema at San Francisco State. (Back then, I dreamt of being a film auteur like Kubrick, Billy Wilder, or David Fincher.) Walking around our small, idyllic campus at Saint Mary's, being in classes among fellow word nerds who also thirsted and lived to read and write

---

[*] Much later, I came across a study that found that 10 percent of male Hodgkin's lymphoma patients receiving ABVD chemotherapy developed aspermia—the inability to create any semen. It could have been worse, though. The MOPP chemotherapy regimen, a toxic combination of four drugs that used to be the standard treatment for Hodgkin's lymphoma patients until the 1980s, caused 85 percent of male Hodgkin's lymphoma patients to develop aspermia.

good stories was nourishing for my spirit. In Wesley Gibson and Marilyn Abildskov—my nonfiction professors at Saint Mary's—I had found two writing mentors. I felt at home among my classmates and professors. At peace with myself. Throughout my young adulthood, I often felt as if I never quite fit in with any group of people—at least not for long. It had taken *my entire life* to figure out that I was a writer, to figure out that fellow writers *were* my tribe on this earth. I didn't want to be taken from that community.

After our meeting, I stood in line in the hallway to make my next appointment. My social worker, Rachel, walked over. She placed a hand on my shoulder.

"Hey, are you okay?" she asked. She must have seen the hangdog expression on my face.

I sighed deeply.

"I just wanna go home and throw myself on my bed and cry," I said. "Dr. Attali said I should forget about going back to school—that I'm going to be too sick to handle a full class load."

"Well, he's not necessarily right. What if you took fewer classes? Can you do that?"

Like a string puppet, my slouching body raised. My eyes bloomed.

"I think I can. I'll have to ask, but I'm sure they can make an exception for me, given my circumstance."

I took a BART train over to the community center where I worked in West Oakland, across the bay. When the train emerged from the deafening Transbay Tube, I felt like the weather outside—sunlight shining over me in the East Bay, dark-gray fog hovering over San Francisco.

A few days later, I cycled over to the San Francisco Main Library. I looked up books on lymphoma and chemotherapy, and then hoofed up to the fourth floor. When I located the corresponding stack, past the resource desk and communal reading area, I felt hesitant to approach it. A bespectacled librarian manned the resource desk nearby. Other library staff members hovered by. I was afraid one of them would look over at me, standing alone in that section, and know, aha, he must have cancer.

I read up on other possible side effects to look forward to besides chemo classics such as nausea and vomiting and fatigue and hair loss (which I learned could grow back differently—curly when it was straight, coarse when it was smooth, even a different shade depending on the color of the administered chemo. I thought this was kinda cool). They included:

- Diarrhea
- Constipation
- A change in sense of taste and smell (a book recommended that patients keep a set of plastic utensils because it is possible to experience a foul, metallic taste from silverware)
- Sterility
- Bleeding gums
- Mouth sores
- Sensitivity to sunlight (it would be easier to get sunburnt)
- Hyperpigmentation (a darkening of the skin, like freckles)
- Brittle fingernails
- "Chemo brain"[*]
- Blurred vision
- Cord-like veins (otherwise known as "superficial thrombosis"—a clotting of the veins)

No wonder my dread of chemo ballooned like an aggressive malignant tumor.

One of the books suggested that I keep essential items next to my

---

[*] It has taken some time, but "chemo brain" is recognized by the medical field as a legitimate side effect from certain chemotherapy drugs. *Everyone's Guide to Cancer Survivorship: A Road Map for Better Health*, a guide written by a panel of physicians, states that this effect causes both short- and long-term memory problems for patients receiving such treatment. The American Cancer Society's webpage lists other cognitive problems attributed to chemo brain:

- Trouble concentrating—patients can't focus on what they're doing
- Trouble remembering details like names, dates, and sometimes larger events
- Trouble multitasking, like answering the phone while cooking without losing track of either task
- Trouble remembering common words—an inability to finish a sentence because one can't find the right words

Doctors are unsure of why chemotherapy can cause such cognitive problems. The American Cancer Society website also states that after imaging tests of some patients' brains, the parts correlated to memory, planning, and putting thoughts into action are *smaller* after chemotherapy.

bed—such as water, medications, and snacks my stomach could handle—during treatment because I *should expect* to be sick and bedridden the *days* following an infusion. Reading this made me grimace, like when I read Lucy Grealy's memoir, *Autobiography of a Face*, for my first creative nonfiction class in grad school. In her memoir, Grealy described "the days of vomiting" she suffered after her infusions, how she kept a plastic basin in her bedroom to puke in so she wouldn't have to scamper to the bathroom to retch, and how her veins became so tight from the infusions that it took the nurses three to five sticks to find one that could handle an IV.

I imagined my experience would be similar. Summer would be a miserable, lonely, vomity existence. I imagined I would feel too weak to roll out of bed to trudge down the hall to yack in the toilet. I imagined my weekends would be largely spent on my bed, staring at the white ceiling with a queasy stomach and a basin by my bedside so I could turn to it and vomit. I imagined I would become quite expert at that: projectile vomiting. And my room would perpetually smell like a mixture of puke and 409 cleaner.

To boot, my chemotherapy regimen—Adriamycin, bleomycin, vinblastine, and dacarbazine—didn't *sound* healing. Not one fucking bit. Dacarbazine and Adriamycin, better known as doxorubicin, sounded like toxins you're supposed to be *kept away from,*[*] like industrial pollutants that could fuck up even Superman (*oh no, Superman, look out, its doxorubicin!*), let alone a puny mortal like me.

[*] Up until the early 1980s, mustard gas was one of the primary ingredients used in chemotherapy to treat Hodgkin's lymphoma. (How you'd like to read *that* warning label?) The inception of chemotherapy began during World War II, when military doctors discovered that soldiers exposed to mustard gas were killed because their bone marrow was decimated. During autopsies, it was found that these casualties had lower white blood cell counts. And so, the proverbial light bulb clicked on, and in 1942 U.S. doctors put mustard gas's anticancerous properties to the test by using "nitrogen mustard" to treat lymphoma, according to Cancer Research UK. The drug was administered intravenously because they found that it was too irritating to inhale the gas.

The treatments were not very successful.

Fight

TWO MONTHS BEFORE I got the Bad News, I went online and found a black-and-white photo of a Cuban boxer standing in a boxing ring. The chiseled, dark-skinned boxer was unrecognizable, his face cloaked in shadow. By then, I feared I had a blood cancer. And so, I decided to accept my potential fight with lymphoma as just that: a fight. A battle. A war. The last thing I wanted was to be caught flat-footed, thumped against the ropes, left in a daze from the wallop that *CANCER* packs.

After I was diagnosed, I stared at the picture on occasion, which I had saved to my computer. I had bought wholesale into Western medicine's warlike approach toward cancer, so I worked toward seeing myself as a fighter. I began to imagine my fight with Mr. Hodgkins as an epic death match—as though we were angels clashing swords high up in the clouds, dramatic string movements ringing in the air. (This is what I pictured when I listened to Metallica's performance of "The Call of Ktulu" with the San Francisco Symphony Orchestra.) Though it wasn't a conscious tactic at first, I listened to more and more hard, fast, violent music from my iPod when I cycled to and from school, or to the hospital for my pre-chemo examinations—old-school thrash metal from Metallica and my cherished fuck-you punk rock by bands such as the Sex Pistols, Dead Kennedys, and Pateando Tu Kara (a fierce punk band from Lima, Peru). This was my fight music. No one—no punk-ass, deathmonger motherfucker was going to take me down without a nasty, nasty fight.

During the lead-up to chemo, I watched Brian De Palma's *Scarface* for the first time since I was fourteen. I became enamored—as I always had been—by the bloody shootout at the end of the film, where a coked-out

Tony Montana shoots it out with a slew of guerilla soldiers that invade his mansion. But now that I was in this aggressive fight mode, I became fixated with that scene; I YouTubed it again and again. I twisted it into a lymphoma-inspired remake in which I starred as Tony Montana, standing on the balcony with an assault rifle in my hands.

C'mon! Who you think you're fucking with, man? I'm Juan Alvarado Valdivia! You fuck with me, you fuckin' with the best!

The soldiers below, cowering behind bullet-ridden walls, ducking along the stairwells, are Mr. Hodgkins's clones—middle-aged men in black suits with derby hats. After I take a few slugs, cackling, *C'mon! Is that all ya got?* I mow them down with the rifle, *bangbangbangbangbangbangbang*, blood splattering on the walls, bodies crumbling to the ground. The bullets I beg for (*C'mon!*) are the ill effects I will receive from chemo. The key difference between my adaptation and De Palma's film is that I am left standing.

SEE YOU ALL IN FUCKIN' HELL! I would shout, holding the smoking assault rifle as I looked down upon the corpses of Mr. Hodgkins strewn all over the mansion, their blood congealing into the carpet.

A Day in the Life of Mr. Hodgkins

INT. JUAN'S MEDIASTINUM—DAY

In a cavern within the tumor just over Juan Alvarado Valdivia's heart, Mr. Hodgkins has his loafers kicked up on his polished executive desk. He is a pudgy, light-skinned man in his mid-fifties. He wears a white button-down shirt, red tie, and vest beneath his black tuxedo jacket. He leans back in his black leather chair with a carefree grin, his hands clasped behind his head. His derby hat is slanted forward.

A soldier, one of Hodgkins's minions, walks into his lair. He brings a steaming cup of dark coffee on a silver tray.

SOLDIER
Your coffee, sir.

He places it on the desk next to a tidy stack of papers.

MR. HODGKINS
Thank you, thank you.

Mr. Hodgkins tips his hat back into place and sits forward to reach the cup. The soldier stands erect at the foot of his desk. Mr. Hodgkins takes a long guzzle of his coffee.

SOLDIER
Sir—

Mr. Hodgkins puts his cup down. He looks up at the soldier with steely eyes.

MR. HODGKINS
 Yes?

SOLDIER
 Um, sir—what should we do today?

Mr. Hodgkins yawns, opens a drawer, and pulls out a dart. He leans back in his chair, kicking his feet up on the desk. He looks over at the far wall, which has a life-size cutout of Juan's internal body hanging from it. A dart is piercing the heart.

MR. HODGKINS
 What we do every day, soldier—kill, kill, kill.

He throws the dart. It pierces Juan's forehead with a thunk.

SOLDIER
 Sir, yes sir.

MR. HODGKINS
 Tell your commanding officer to continue to concentrate our forces on spreading to his vital organs.

SOLDIER
 Sir, yes sir.

The soldier salutes him with a knife hand before leaving. Mr. Hodgkins reaches again into the drawer. He holds a dart by his right eye, squinting with his other as he eyes the dartboard.

MR. HODGKINS
 Your days are numbered, sonny boy.

Mr. Hodgkins rears his arm and throws another dart.

The Big Jizz Decision

ONE MORNING, WITH the sun lighting our flat, I walked down the hall as my roommate, Kelly, sat in our living room. He was writing on his laptop. By then, I had shorn off my hair to preempt the chemo. Like the Incan warrior who leapt off a tower to his death rather than surrender to the conquistadors during a battle at Sacsayhuamán in 1536, I didn't want to allow the chemotherapy drugs to have the power to take my hair.

"Hey, Juan, have you decided if you're storing your sperm?" he asked.

"Not yet," I said from my bedroom. "I still have to check their pricing."

By then, during my last gulps of Life Before Chemo, I had finally turned to that printout from the Sperm Bank of California. In the frequently asked questions section, I read: "Between 50% to 80% of sperm die in the freezing process." What a tough gig it is to be a sperm, I thought. When introduced into a fertile female, millions of them don't reach the top of the mountain, so to speak. Even in the freeze-and-tuck-you-away-just-in-case-I-need-you game of sperm storage, most of my procreative puppies would die.

The handout and the Sperm Bank of California's website had these other fun facts and answers:

- "Frozen semen can be stored for as long as 50 years without additional sperm deterioration." (Deterioration?)
- "Sperm samples are stored in tanks of liquid nitrogen, which must be kept at -196 degrees Celsius or -321 degrees Fahrenheit." (Rats! I knew I couldn't just toss them in our freezer.)

- "Can I provide samples at home? As soon as you ejaculate, the sperm in your ejaculate begins to deteriorate. We ask that you provide your semen samples on our premises so our lab can begin the cryopreservation process as soon as possible. . . ." (What kind of whack-off material do they provide at their office?)

After I told Kelly I had not checked the sperm bank's pricing, I could hear a flurry of keystrokes from the living room. He was looking it up. A minute later, he shouted, "Hey Juan! It's gonna cost you seven hundred to set it up. Three fifty every other year."

And so, the decision to not cryogenically freeze my seed was simple. It cost too much.

The Sperm Bank of California charged "client depositors" (men storing semen for spouse or intimate partner) $350 for an "initial semen storage visit/consultation." In addition, there was an annual fee of $350 for "semen storage and handling." At that clip, the first year of storage—or sperm parking, as I preferred to call it—would total $700. Each subsequent year would cost $350.

It cost too much for too many hypotheticals involved—*if* the sperm samples survived, *if* they could even impregnate this hypothetical future partner, *if* chemo would make me impotent, *if* I even wanted children someday.

Sperm storage seemed like a risky luxury I didn't want to afford. Plus, my altruistic side was quite open to adoption. Nonetheless, I dreaded sharing this decision with my parents.

A few days later, on the last weekend of May, I went to Fremont for a family barbecue. Carmen was in town, but my main purpose in visiting was to share my decision with our parents.

They were in the backyard when I walked through the living room. Through the sliding glass door, I saw my dad standing behind the grill with barbecue tongs in hand. He was chatting with Heide, who was drinking a Corona. My mom was placing her boom box and a handful of her CDs on a foldout table. She was alone. It was my opportunity. Looking down at the mahogany floor, I went over all the reasons I had for not freezing my sperm, in case she responded with disappointment and asked me why. I opened the screen door and walked toward her until she turned to me.

"Ma," I said, my voice low.

"Sí, mijo," she said with an expectant tone.

My head was slouched while I faced her. I looked off to the side, hesitant to look into her eyes, as though I was a boy who knew he had done something wrong.

"You know about—how I have to decide if I'm freezing my sperm?"

"Sí."

"I decided not to. I did some research—and it just costs too much."

"Oh, don't worry about it. Like I told you before, my coworker's husband had testicular cancer. He had one of them removed, and now they're married and have two kids."

Phew.

Nevertheless, I was taken aback by her nonchalant response. She was certain that my reproductive system would be just as vigorous after chemotherapy.

At the time, I almost felt charmed that the matter of someday fertilizing my own children was out of my hands. It was as though it was up to the cosmos if my blood would carry on.

In a way, it seemed beautiful.

But what if the chemo *would* make me sterile?

What if I ever had a partner who was adamant about having my children?

My Last Weekend before Liftoff to Toxic-Puke-Retch Land

FRIDAY NIGHT, THE first weekend of June, I was riding shotgun in Paola's car while she drove us out of the Mission. Her roommate, Lizette, sat in the back wearing a dress that hardly concealed her bountiful chest. We were all dressed up, riding over to a club near the Panhandle.

The week before, I met with Dr. Attali to go over the results of my recent examinations. My ticker was good. My lungs were "unremarkable," which meant they were normal. In addition to my chemotherapy being green-lighted, the PET scan showed that the cancerous mass over my heart measured 6.8 cm × 2.1 cm. About the size of a meatball or a Super Ball. In Attali's opinion, the tumor was just big enough that radiation treatment was recommended after chemo was over. I would have to meet with his mentor, Dr. Kirsch—a man he revered—at UCSF's renowned Radiation Oncology Department to explore that treatment option.

When Friday, June 5, rolled around—when it dawned on me that it was the final weekend before liftoff to Toxic-Puke-Retch Land—I wished I was far away. I wished I was doing something super special. I wished I was with my cousins in a smoky discotheque in Arequipa getting sauced up on pisco, our words all slurry, arms around one another. Or at a beach in Cambodia, lying in a hammock, the sky swabbed in orange sunset. Or riding my bicycle, Blue, beneath towering pine trees in Yosemite Valley with El Capitan in the distance. Once I was undergoing chemotherapy, I wasn't sure how much I would be able to physically do. I was afraid it could be the last weekend I would have for some time in which I would feel *normal*. Myself—100 percent moi. Not chemo-me—a weaker, lesser version of myself.

But once I realized the gravity of that first weekend in June, it was too late to make any big plans. So when Paola invited me to go dancing with her friends, I gladly accepted. Dancing had already crossed my mind. I could see myself dancing alone in a throng of people, numbly drunk, my eyes closed, my head swaying from side to side, my body lost in communion with the pulsing music. When I pictured it, it felt cleansing. Something defiant, something bittersweet, something joyous.

When we rolled up to the club, there was a long line of stylishly dressed youngsters waiting outside. That's when I remembered that I wasn't particularly fond of clubs. I had somehow forgotten in the midst of my dance-cleanse daydream.

Paola slowed the car, searching for a spot. I looked at the line and huffed.

"I am *not* standing in that line," I said.

"We don't have to stand at the end of the line," Paola said, turning the corner. "Stephanie should already be waiting for us."

While we looked for parking, I took out my wallet to ensure I had exact fare for the bus. My "Plan B." I could always abort the mission.

By the time we got to the front door, Paola's friend, Stephanie, was near the front of the line. We hardly waited, but I was still upset. I felt trapped, far from home, far from nightspots I dug, ones that weren't scenes for douchy people like the kind this club appeared to attract. I also felt a strain pressing against the sides of my head: *I have to have a really great time. I have to have a really great time.* I felt a desperate pressure to make the night count.

That pressure came closer to boiling when the doorman asked for a $10 cover charge. I was tempted to say *fuck this*, but we had gone all the way there. And I didn't want to let Paola down. So I hoped for the best, paid, and went in with them.

I regretted that decision within minutes.

We stood in the main room, close to the DJ. We had to lean close and shout into each other's ears just to hear what we were saying. The pressure in my head kept building like the sound of the screeching subway train growing when Michael Corleone shot those guys in an Italian restaurant in *The Godfather*.

While Paola talked with her friends, I stomped off without saying a word. I zigzagged through the crowd to the bar. Luckily, no one bumped into me, because I had my I-could-not-give-a-fuck face on. The minutes passed slowly as I waited and waited at the counter, standing on my tippy-toes in hopes of getting one of the bartenders' attention. I saw Paola at the end of the crowded bar. She probably figured I should be left alone. A bartender finally got to me. I ordered a shot and a gin and tonic. I downed the shot, set the empty glass firmly on the bar, and took the gin and tonic with me as I rejoined Paola and her crew.

We continued to stand in the middle of the room. The DJ was playing loud, atrocious hip-hop to a room full of people who were not dancing.

"I don't get it," I said, shouting into Paola's ear. "Did everyone get out of their house and pay ten dollars to come here to stand around and shout into each other's ears just to have a conversation?"

She grinned nervously. I crossed my arms. My drink was going down *way* too fast.

A minute later, Lizette suggested that we step into the back room where they had the main dance floor. I was relieved. I was hopeful that we could do something besides pick our butts while shouting into each other's ears, but that dark room provided no relief. No one was dancing. It was a little past 10 p.m. The alcohol had not lubricated our limbs into gyration.

I think Paola's friends could sense the tension boiling inside me, because Stephanie began to dance all jokey with her drink in hand. She was trying to lighten the mood. "This is fucking stupid," I said after a while.

We retreated back to the first room. In the hallway between them, I walked beside Paola.

"I'm sorry, but I'm going home," I said to her.

"How?"

"I'll take the bus. Don't worry about it. I knew I should have never come in. You should stay and have fun with your friends. I don't want to ruin your night out."

When we got to the other room, I told Stephanie and Lizette I was leaving. And although I pleaded with her to stay, Paola left her friends to be with me. It was awkward when we left, but I was relieved. The pressure swirling in my head seemed to dissipate once we stepped out into the cool night.

Paola drove us back to the Mission. We went to the Make Out Room, which played salsa on Saturday nights. It was my kind of joint: casual, decent music, not a posh place to be seen. It was a bar we were fond of. I felt bad about what had happened, but I was happy to be alone with her.

After we stepped inside, while waiting at the bar, I turned to Paola. "Why do you put up with me?" I asked.

Paola was taken aback by my question. We stood quiet for a few seconds.

"I don't know," she finally said, which struck me as an honest response.

We were determined to boogie. However, when it comes to dancing, I have a tough time feeling loose and uninhibited unless I'm a bit drunk, so I commenced to get a bit hammered while we sat at the bar. After a few drinks, I told Paolita some things I later felt I shouldn't have, since we'd been out for only three months. I told her I loved cumming inside of her. (We had recently started that once she got on birth control. She told me that I was the first guy she had allowed to cum inside of her, which meant something to me.) I told her that if I could be in a relationship with any of my past girlfriends, I would pick her in a second.

Paola and I shimmied and twirled beneath the streamers that hung from the ceiling. The lights that refracted from the spinning disco ball made the dance floor seem like the inside of a kaleidoscope. When they played some cumbias, we danced hand in hand, our cheeks nearly touching before we took turns twirling beneath one of our outstretched arms. The first few turns were awkward, our arms twisted midair like confused pretzels. It made us crack up.

We spent much of the next day together. We slept in, then lazily lay in bed and snuggled before we cooked omelets for breakfast. Paola asked that I apologize to her friends about the night before, which I had already planned to do.

Paola decided to go to Trader Joe's for a food run. I asked to tag along. Two of the chemotherapy books I read suggested having someone who could buy groceries in case I was too weak to do it myself. But I really wanted to go because it felt so couple-like to buy groceries together. And it was, especially when we walked through the sliding automatic doors with one shopping cart. Though I didn't fully realize it then, it was a big deal to me to walk in beside Paola with *our* shopping cart. A supermarket run had been a rare occurrence with any of my previous girlfriends. That image of domesticity—two of us, one shopping cart—was one I had longed for much of my life.

While Paola walked around the store pushing the cart, picking up items from her shopping list, I wandered around and picked up items—rations—I would need for my war. Microwaveable spinach and mushroom quiche, soyrizo, lentil vegetable soup, carrots, WestSoy milk, and chocolate-chip granola bars. Like the books suggested, I jotted these items down. Later, when I handed Paola my shopping list, it felt like an important act for me. It has always been difficult for me to ask help of others. Handing her the list was like an admission of possible weakness on my part. It felt like I was placing myself in her hands.

Out in the parking lot, Paolita and I walked side by side as I pushed our cart to her car. A cover of clouds hung over Daly City, concealing the sun as a cool breeze blew. I smiled as I looked over at her. I felt so grateful to have found a partner who would support me through the most trying period of my life.

The Growl

A FEW DAYS before I began chemotherapy, I came home from a day at work and school. In my bedroom, alit in waning sunlight, I peeled off my office getup. My roommates weren't home. I loved having the flat to myself so I could blast a danceable tune or some rock 'n' roll that was born to be loud. Sometimes I would roar to the song, bang my head, even bust out some air-guitar flails. I flipped through my spinning CD tower. Metallica's ferocious cover of Diamond Head's "Am I Evil?" was what I felt pulsing in my veins. I needed some induced catharsis.

An unexpected thing happened while I stood there listening to the militaristic intro blare through the flat. Like a howling wolf, I craned my head back and roared in the hopes of letting out some of the frustration I had been feeling from Life with Lymphoma, especially after I had had to subject myself to a second bone marrow biopsy a few days before. The joyous, playful roar that usually came out whenever I would shout along with a rock song was more of an angry, guttural growl. It rattled from my chest and up my throat, filling the room. It felt like something with its own life. Something I couldn't quite control.

And that's when I got a *sense* that I was like a walking human volcano. Beneath the surface, beneath my stoic, I'm-being-strong veneer, the tension was building. Bubbling, rumbling, escalating. It was all those hospital visits. Medical examinations. Agonizing lines to wait in. All that time lost in those drab, life-sucking waiting rooms. All those medical terms and the cancer jargon I had to become familiar with. All those big decisions I had to make: Should I get a catheter port inserted into my arm for the duration of treatment? *Should* I have my sperm frozen? And all the e-mails I had to respond to from my family in Peru, telling me that they were sorry—that I just had to put my faith in God. That this "nightmare" would soon pass. All the times I had to tell them, "It's going to be okay."

As if I really knew.

Round One at 4C

THE NIGHT BEFORE my first infusion, I stayed up past 2 a.m. I sat at my computer, wired with nervous, pace-the-room energy, zipping from webpage to webpage, watching a slew of YouTube videos, including replay after replay of Buster Douglas's famous tenth-round knockout of Mike Tyson.

After I was diagnosed, I became obsessed with the 1990 fight—one of the biggest upsets in sports history. Coming into that fight, Douglas was a 42–1 underdog to Iron Mike, who was seemingly invincible with a 37–0 record that included thirty-three knockouts. By beating Tyson, Douglas rose to the stature of a modern-day giant slayer. In preparing to fight for my life, I watched that knockout countless times—Buster's repeated jabs to Tyson's face in the middle of the ring, luring him closer before he wound his right hand back to deliver a vicious uppercut that snapped Tyson's head back and sent his eyes rolling back in their sockets before Douglas put him down with a quick left-right-left combination, the crowd in Tokyo gasping, witnesses to the unfathomable, the ringside commentator shouting, "Look at this! He's knocked Mike Tyson DOWN! For the first time in his career, Mike Tyson hits the canvas!" Although I had become familiar with the knockout, knew exactly what would happen, I still felt an electric jolt course through me that Thursday night, my eyes welling with tears while I watched Tyson crawl on his knees beside the ropes, his mouth agape as he reached for his mouthpiece before staggering to his feet at the count of nine, the referee clutching him to his chest while he waved the fight off, the bell ringing, crowd roaring, the commentator screaming, "Unbelievable! Unbelievable! *Unbelievable!*"

My life had become remarkably simple at that moment: there was nothing, *absolutely nothing* I wanted more than to be like Buster Douglas on that night in Tokyo, Japan—his arms raised victorious, exhausted and overwhelmed at what he had accomplished.

The morning fog had burned off as I walked out of the house to my parents' green SUV parked on the corner. I sat in the backseat and muttered hello, tired and cranky from the lack of sleep. They wanted to be with me during my first—our first—infusion. My mom was leaving for Peru in two days to care for my grandmother. She would be gone for nearly two months. This was the one infusion she would be able to witness for some time.

We rode down 22nd Street. Ahead, small and faint in the distance, were the tall brick buildings of the San Francisco General campus. The sun shone over the neighborhood. The radio was tuned to my favorite station, 98.1 KISS FM. Their morning DJ wished everyone a happy Friday before he took a request. On Mission Street, people walked to and fro, going about their daily trajectories. It was just another day for most folks. A half hour earlier, in my bedroom, while I packed my bag for treatment—an apple, a banana, Saunders's *CivilWarLand in Bad Decline*, a notebook, and my three pill bottles of nausea medicine—I became incredulous that this moment was actually happening. *Me? Chemofuckingtherapy?* But as we neared the hospital, I became excited. If I had it my way, I would've started chemo right after I got the Bad News. I was finally fighting back.

At 4C—San Francisco General's infusion ward run entirely by nurses—my mom and dad stood beside me in the hallway outside the main infusion room. It was a large room that probably used to be two; half of a wall appeared to have been removed to connect them. The walls were painted in a shade of light green that felt like it was meant to be calming. Two reclining chairs faced the hallway with six others scattered along the walls. At the far end were windows that spanned the entire length of the room. It provided a view of the surrounding city: the hospital's parking garage, the 101 freeway with its ceaseless flow of vehicles that looked like Micro Machines. In the distance, houses dotted the Bernal Heights hillside, the big blue sky draped behind it.

I had been in the ward twice before. On both occasions, I was a bit shocked to find that the doors leading into the infusion room were always open. Anyone could walk by, peer in, and see Cancer Club patients reclined in those chairs with IVs pricked into their arms, mouths gaping open, and eyes shut, zonked out from their meds. When my eyes would meet another patient's, I would turn away. It felt like an intrusion. It felt wrong to be able to see other patients receiving chemotherapy—a treatment *our lives depended on*. It was too intimate to see people at such a vulnerable moment in their lives. Before I visited the infusion ward, I imagined that such an act would be treated more privately, with each patient having their own room. Or behind closed doors at the very least. I didn't think we would be put in a communal salvation room.

We waited until Shannon, one of the nurses, led us in. It was easy to remember her name; she reminded me of actress/comedian Molly Shannon, only with red highlights and blue eye shadow. I took one of the chairs against a wall. To my left was a view of the outside—the sunshine, the world I desperately wanted to continue to be a part of. On my right were the doors leading into the room, with two identical clocks hanging over the doorways. Shannon took my hospital card, verified my name and date of birth, then left. My parents stood close by without saying a word. They looked around with somber eyes. The reality must have smacked them: Cancer World, now a part of our world.

On our side of the infusion room were three other patients. A woman lay on a hospital bed next to the big window. The morning sun bathed her in soft light while she slept on her side. The other patients sat in their chairs. They were eyeing us—the rookies. They were in their forties or early fifties. I was the baby there.

Three other nurses zigzagged around the room, attending to their patients. I passed the time by trying to amuse my parents with some shabby quips. (For example, "I think they're trying to confuse us, since *that* clock is a few seconds ahead of that one," I said, pointing to the clock over the doorway closest to us. Much later, when my parents were getting ready to leave to grab some food at Walgreens, I joked with my dad about the unlikelihood of getting a pizza delivered to the ward.) I felt obligated to entertain them since they were just standing there. Being the jester had been my self-assigned role in our family for so long, especially after my sisters left home and I stayed. For years, until I moved out when I was twenty-five, I felt it was my duty to keep things fun and light between my parents. I felt it was my responsibility to make them happy.

Before long, we heard a "ding-dong, ding-dong" sound from the other end of the room. It was the kind of sound a car makes when a door is left open. We watched one of the nurses race toward it. She bent over a weird-looking machine. Every patient had one, including me. It looked like a rolling parking meter with a number pad. The machine—an infusion pump—was connected to the drip bag that hung above the man laid out on a reclining chair. The nurse clicked a few buttons on the machine to cease the beeping.

Soon afterward, a middle-aged black nurse walked over to me. She was chewing gum, which made her seem relaxed yet authoritative, like a yard duty. Tucked against her side was a green file. She held an array of wrapped, sterilized supplies.

"Hi Juan, my name is Marva," she said in an accent that sounded Caribbean. "I'm going to be your nurse today."

I smiled and said hi. She greeted my parents.

"All right. While we wait for the pharmacy to prepare your medicine, let's get you started. Which arm do you want?"

It was a question I had already considered.

Thought about *a lot.*

For chemotherapy itself, the key decision I had to make was if I should get a catheter port installed. The catheter—a thin, flexible tube—would be inserted in a vein beneath one of my arms, then threaded into a large vein in the chest. It would simplify things for the nurses since they could draw blood and inject chemo through a port that the catheter would be connected to. This way, they wouldn't have to poke a needle into my arms for every infusion or blood draw. The only drawback was I would have this port installed in my body for the duration of treatment, which could be four to six months. Also, since it could get infected, the port required vigilant cleaning.

I opted not to get it installed. Though I had no previous experience to gather from, I figured chemo wouldn't be so bad on my arms. Plus, I was hopeful that I would only have to do a minimum of eight infusions—maybe one or two more. I was afraid that people would notice the catheter port and rightly deduce that something was wrong with me. One of my key strategies in handling cancer was to try and go about my life as normally as possible. But more importantly, I was afraid it would appear unattractive to Paola. That it would taint something as beautiful, as peaceful as the feeling I had when we were in each other's arms. I didn't want that intimacy to be tarnished.

But in time, the chemo *was* going to mess up my veins. My poor veins would not appreciate the harsh treatment, and they would tighten up and "hide"—as the nurses at 4C put it. They would darken and clot, become difficult to draw blood from. In a sense, Marva was asking, "Which arm do you wanna fuck up?"

"My left arm," I said (since I'm right-handed).

Marva lifted the chair arm on my left side. She pulled a stool over and sat on it. While humming a tune, she unwrapped a sterilizing wipe, butterfly needle, and adhesives that would keep my IV in place. She grabbed a large blue rubber band and tied it tight behind my elbow.

My parents inched closer. Especially my mother. She was practically hovering over Marva, staring at her handiwork as she stuck the needle into my forearm. (Before she married my dad, my mom was studying to be a nurse in Peru. She was a semester away from graduating before they moved to Mexico.) I shot a stern look at my parents. Their concerned eyes were like glaring spotlights. It would have made me apprehensive if I were Marva. To avoid glaring at my parents, I looked off at the wall.

Just go away. There's nothing you can do. You don't have to worry. I'm in good hands.

Marva connected my IV to a bag of saline. Its function was to dilute my bloodstream so my veins could handle the chemo. Once she left the room, I bent over the side of the chair to grab my shoulder bag from the ground. My father stepped over as fast as he could to help.

"I got it, Dad," I said in a voice that made him halt. He stood frozen for a second before he stepped back to my mother, like I had disciplined him.

I reached inside my bag to grab a highlighter and *CivilWarLand in Bad Decline*. I tried extra hard to zoom in on every line to block my parents from my peripheral vision. Since I was their son—my body, my life, in a way, just as much theirs—I felt I couldn't tell them to leave. I didn't want to banish them to the ward's cold, dreary waiting room. At the same time, I didn't know what to say to them to pass the time.

Watching over me, keeping me company seemed like the only way they could care for me. Neither of them are conversationalists, especially my father, who has always been a quiet, modest man. (During meals, it's typical for him to not say much besides, "Can you pass the bread?" He gets chatty when he's tipsy, which is a rare occurrence.) I know they felt powerless, but they were taxing me. Even though I had not asked them to be with me during my infusion, I couldn't help but feel like a burden to them.

Marva, bless her, never told my parents to wait outside (though, eventually, they did when more patients filed into the infusion room). I'm sure she could have, but she didn't. A few months later, she would tell me about her kids during one of my infusions.

She must have known, better than I had, how my parents felt at that moment.

About two hours after we showed up for treatment, Shannon walked into the ward. She held a large Ziploc-like bag. "Alvarado. I've got Alvarado's chemo," she said aloud.

She dropped the bag off on my armrest. Marva walked over.

"Can you do a chemo check?" Marva asked her.

"Give me a minute. I need to check on one of my patients," Shannon said, before they zipped away. They came back a minute later. Marva stepped to my right side and lifted my arm.

"Your name and date of birth?" Shannon asked.

"Juan Alvarado. Four, four, seventy-nine," I said while Marva held up my arm to read the name and DOB stamped on my yellow hospital wristband. Shannon opened the bag, which had a big yellow-and-black logo of three intertwined circles in its middle. It looked like the sign you see in movies or TV shows for toxic materials or hazardous areas. Below that sign it read:

CAUTION
Chemotherapy/Cytotoxic
Material.
After Use, Dispose of in
Accordance with
Established Procedure

I could feel myself squirm inside. They were going to inject that shit *in me*, not keep me from it. If I were an old-school Looney Tunes character, my eyes would have bulged before I gave a big gulp.

"This is for Alvarado, Juan. Medical record number 017*****," Shannon said, holding up a paper that was folded in the bag. The equivalent of a packing list, I presumed. (*Let's see what we got ourselves here. Shit that will fuck you up, aaaannd . . . some more shit that will fuck you up.*) Marva muttered the first numbers and released my arm.

"I have Benadryl, twenty-five," Shannon said, pulling out a pill tablet from the bag.

"Benadryl, twenty-five," Marva said, holding up my patient file, scribbling on a paper.

"Anzemet, ten. Tylenol and Ativan."

"Anzemet, ten. Tylenol—Ativan."

"Bleomycin, eighteen, push." Shannon pulled out a syringe—minus the needle—containing a clear liquid. "And then I have a test dose for a total of 19."

They continued on, verifying the contents. Then Marva handed me a form.

"Just sign here at the bottom, to consent to your treatment," she said. She pointed a pen at the "client/representative signature" line near the bottom of the form.

I was bewildered from their chemo check—how orderly and borderline militaristic it was. I appreciated that they were ensuring I was the right person getting the right treatment and the right dosages, but it just reinforced how deadly serious this all was. Marva's business-is-business tone when she asked me to sign the form perturbed me further. The warmth her voice exuded before was gone, which is partly why my bullshit detector awoke with a jolt. Since I was signing a form, I was inclined to read it to make sure I wasn't getting reamed. But then I remembered—ha!—that *I would be* fucked if I didn't have treatment. Like, my-dead-ass-in-the-ground screwed. (Would the Kama Sutra name such a position "The Necrophiliac's Delight"?) There was no sense in reading it before signing. Shit, I was beyond fortunate to have this life-saving treatment available to me—and for free through the city's health plan.

I signed.

Soon after, Marva gave me a cup of water and a teeny pill cup. It held Tylenol and Ativan pills that would help with nausea. Fifteen minutes after I gulped them, my head felt light and woozy. I whipped my head to the sides. Everything blurred. My eyelids felt heavy. Before I ever had chemo, I had vowed to myself that I would not be like the other patients. I would not allow myself to pass out like them, curled up in a bed, stretched out in a reclining chair. I would read through my infusions or entertain myself somehow. I told myself I had too much fight, too much gusto to zonk out from my treatments. Now I know that I just didn't want to look so vulnerable and weak.

Despite the wooziness, I continued to read. Marva took a seat on the stool beside me, just as my mom dropped by for one of her cameos from the waiting room.

"All right, we're going to give you this test dosage first," Marva said, connecting one of the chemo "push" syringes to my IV. "We do it to make sure you don't have an allergic reaction to it."

With my book held open, I watched her gently push the drug into my IV out of the corner of my eye. My mom stood to my right, her back to the wall. Her face contorted into a harrowing, resigned look. It was the same expression she had when she held our dog, Cotton, in her arms when we took him to be put down. Except this time, her eyes were tearing. (A few weeks after I was diagnosed, I talked on the phone with her. I was giving her an update on all the pre-chemo examinations I had to do. Near the end of our call, she started to cry. She told me in Spanish, "I just can't stand to see you sick, to see you have to suffer. I wish I could be the one who was sick so I could take all the pain.") I looked over at her and tried to make a stoic face.

On her way out of the ward, Shannon walked past my mother.

"Don't cry. He's going to be all right," she said, rubbing her arm.

Two hours later, round one was in the bag. The clocks above the doorway read a little past one. After Marva bandaged my arm, I bent over to grab my shoes. For a moment, my torso felt like it was going to tip over, like a falling tree. I slipped on my shoes while my parents stood nearby, watching. I stood up, steadied myself, then wobbled past them to the bathroom. Sweet baby Jesus, I had to go. I'd been holding it in all day, afraid to get up and move around while I was hooked to the IV. To my perverse delight, my urine came out looking like pink lemonade from the red tint of the doxorubicin (which looked like Kool-Aid in its syringe). I washed my hands and peered at my reflection. *That wasn't so bad. I don't feel great, but I don't feel like complete shit.*

On my way out, I said bye to Marva. My parents walked on either side of me down the hallway.

"You look pale," my mother said. She looked concerned.

"Really?"

"Yeah. A little."

We walked out of the hospital to the drop-off rotunda in front. The entire Mission District opened before us. The sun shone over the neighborhood as if it were saying "ta-da!"

"Do you want to wait here while we get the car, son?" my father asked.

"No, I'm fine," I said. Usually such a question about my physical ability would have irritated me, because it seemed clear that I could manage to walk one single block to his Toyota Rav4. But it'd been a long morning on us. I still felt dim and sluggish from the nausea medication.

We walked in silence. A faint breeze whistled. I stared at my feet. Not because I felt sorry for myself, but because I was afraid I might suddenly lose my balance and fall forward.

My parents and I sat at a table in the middle of Taqueria San Francisco, sipping horchatas with a sense of collective relief. The chemo had not walloped me, didn't immediately turn me into a puking machine. Later that afternoon, I'd take a long nap on my parents' couch with Negrita, Heide's black cat. She slept beside me, tucked against my tummy. (Negrita was practically *our* cat since she preferred to stay at our home after we took care of her during one of Heide's vacations. She would become my chemo buddy. After most of my infusions, I'd come home and often pass out on the couch for hours, spooning Negrita.) The next morning, I would awaken in my old bedroom with a wrenching hunger. To my great fortune and complete surprise, this was the most noticeable effect I would observe from my first infusion.

I looked out the taqueria windows. I was hoping to spot one of my ex-roommates walking by. Taqueria San Francisco was a joint I frequented when I lived at my first home in the city, a.k.a. the Bros House.[*]

[*] That's how Paola and I referred to the punk-rock household in the dirty Mission District that I shared with three roommates I met through Craigslist. There was Herman

The first time I ate at the taqueria was five years before on a cloudless Sunday afternoon. I sat next to the windows. I stared out onto 24th Street, watching all the people walking, cycling, or skateboarding by. Across the street, a line formed at St. Francis Fountain, a diner established back in 1918. I had just gone over to my soon-to-be-new home to give my roommate, Robbie, my deposit and first month's rent. He gave me a key to the house and welcomed me with a firm hug and a few hits from his joint. I left in giddy spirits. I was finally moving out of my parents' house—moving to the city, to a vibrant neighborhood, to a household with cool-ass roommates. For the first time in a long time, I felt as if I was exactly where I should be.

At one point—perhaps because I was high—I began to freak out as I stared out onto the corner of 24th and York. I'm moving *here*, I thought. It was so different, bustling with life. Back in Fremont, I stepped out of the house to our yawn of a suburban neighborhood where hardly anyone ever walked on the sidewalks. Here there were people zipping to and fro. But that wave of panic soon passed. I bit into my burrito and grinned as I stared out at the barrio I couldn't wait to become a part of.

Five years later (in one of life's bizarre twists), I found myself back at Taqueria San Francisco with my parents after my first chemotherapy infusion. My greasy burrito was just as good as it had always been there, but I savored it more being there with my parents. Mi mama would take off in two days to be with our family in Peru. I knew she felt torn between being with me—her only son—through the entirety of my treatment or with her mother. Mi abuelita was mostly alone at the home they had always lived in. Each year, she grew more and more senile. Although I wanted her to stay so she could care for me if I got ill, I told my mother she should be with mi abuelita. Mama Carmen

---

(a.k.a. Chaos, a.k.a. DJ Chaos, a.k.a. Chiflas—Spanish for "whistling" since he liked to do just that to chicks with pretty faces or punk-rock floosies), Roberto (a.k.a. Robbie, a.k.a. DJ Tozz Grave), and Ace (a.k.a. Hace Frio, a.k.a. Ace of Spades). Our flat was like a post-frat pad with a dash of Vegas (when I interviewed for the vacant room, Robbie—with the Clash's *London Calling* poster hanging behind him, said there was one house rule: "What happens in this house, stays in this house"), heavy dabs of punk rock, Latino ska, and reggae/rocksteady to accompany the clouds of Maria Jane that swirled around the turntables in our living room. Their friends dubbed our house Casa Pacheco. *Pacheco* is Mexican slang for "stoned," which is what we often were in that house, mostly due to the resplendent amount of marijuana that Robbie smoked every day and almost always shared with whomever was around (like me!).

was in her early nineties. I told my mom we would have plenty of years to be together (or so I needed to believe), but we couldn't be sure about mi abuelita.

In the meantime, I was so grateful to be graced with this moment: lunch with my parents on a sunny afternoon in the city I loved at a taqueria I could point at and say, "*That's* my place."

How Cancer and Chemotherapy Apparently Made Me Homicidal

TWO DAYS AFTER my infusion, my dad drove us to San Francisco Airport to drop off my mom for her trip. When he parked at the terminal curb, I hopped out to help unload her two hefty suitcases.[*] I pulled out the heaviest one—probably a good sixty pounds—with my left arm. A dagger of pain shot from the crook of my arm when I lifted it to the curb. My left forearm had felt a little tender from where they injected the chemo.

After my mom checked in her bags, my dad and I saw her off at the security checkpoint. She was stoic when we hugged and kissed goodbye.

"Cuidate mucho mijito," she said with urgency, rubbing my shoulder. "And please look after your father."

"I will, Ma."

I could sense that it was difficult for her to leave me at that precarious moment in our lives. (Later, she would tell me that she cried once she sat on the plane.) It made me feel sad, somewhere inside, when my dad and I turned to leave.

Four days later, bags under my eyes, nerves all frayed, I cycled over to San Francisco General. I had called the oncology nurse the day before

---

[*] Among our family, my mom is notorious for packing suitcases that would make Mr. T break a sweat. Every time she flies to Arequipa—ever since we were kids—she packs *at least* one suitcase stuffed with clothes and shoes for our cousins and aunts and uncles that she bought on sale or at thrift stores. She often pawns off one of these suitcases on me or my sisters when we travel with her. Or without her. Santa Claus has nothing on my mom.

to tell her about the mild but ceaseless burning sensation I had in the crook of my left arm. To fall asleep, I downed shots of hard alcohol in the middle of the long, long night to numb the pain. She told me the 4C nurses would be expecting me.

Boy she wasn't kidding.

When I got to 4C, Shannon spotted me in the hallway outside the infusion room. My shoulder bag was slung over my back, my bike helmet clutched against my side. (Bringing it along with me to my hospital visits was a tactical choice. The gray helmet—which looked like a fighter pilot helmet à la *Top Gun*, with red and blue stripes splitting down its middle and white stars adorning the sides—was quite noticeable. My doctors, caregivers, and fellow cancer patients could see it. I wanted them to know that although I had cancer and was receiving chemotherapy, it wasn't going to keep me from cycling around the city, from trying my darndest to be physically strong.) Before I could explain why I was there, Shannon said, "Please take a seat, Mr. Alvarado." The bubbly light tone she used when I had my infusion a week before was gone. It sounded like I was in trouble.

The bearded oncology Fellow who seemingly botched my first bone marrow biopsy attended to me. He asked me to describe the pain, then asked what happened during my infusion. He took a look at my arm. Noreen, a sweetie of a nurse, stood nearby to see how I was holding up. As I suspected, given the Google searches I had done the day before, the pain in my arm was not due to extravasation—the seepage of chemotherapy into the surrounding tissue. The doctor told me that would have produced a gnarly bruise. The pain would have occurred during infusion—and it would have been *excruciating.* Extravasation can cause permanent tissue damage. Adriamycin—one of my chemotherapy drugs—is so corrosive that it can cause third-degree burns if it is spilled onto one's skin.

The oncology staff could not explain why the crook of my arm felt like it was burning over a low flame. They recommended cold compresses and some ibuprofen. I asked about getting some Vicodin but was told I would have to get a prescription through Dr. Attali. Then I asked if it was all right to drink some booze—say, wine—to comfort me. El doctorcito laughed.

"A glass or two certainly won't kill you while you're undergoing chemotherapy," he said.

We laughed it up. I had mad appreciation for his dark sense of humor—the inclusion of the word "kill" in a conversation with a lymphoma patient *in an infusion ward*. Flashing my hard-luck-kid smirk, I slipped on my bag and see-you-latered out of there. A six-pack of brewskis and Tylenol helped me sleep that night.

Late Friday afternoon, I walked into Tagi's office in the Mission. It was meant to be a drive-by hello since I happened to be in that part of the neighborhood after meeting up with my friend Barbara. Tagi flashed a big grin when she saw me waving to her by the front door. I was dressed in comfy-nerdy clothes: my brand-new blue Saucony shoes, brown slacks, a T-shirt of an exasperated Hostess cupcake jumping rope with a carrot and broccoli, and my beloved blue cardigan (Paola liked to call it the Old Man Sweater; I think that was her passive way of saying that she didn't like it—she preferred it when I dressed like a guy out of a J-Crew ad). She gave me a big hug and asked if I wanted to grab some dinner with her. "Perfect!" I said.

And that's how our mad-drunken odyssey in the Mission began that Friday evening: two pints at Dalva Bar (might have had a shot of Wild Turkey as well), a pitcher of sangria with tapas at Picaro, a pitcher of beer at Bollywood Cafe (might have had a shot, too), and a tamarind rum drink at the Little Baobab dance club before I blacked out at the crowded-ass Beauty Bar.

The next morning, I awoke in my bed wearing the T-shirt and slacks I had worn the night before. I shot up in bed with that familiar uh-oh feeling. Then I saw my shoes scattered on the floor. Beside them was a wooden piece from my IKEA drawer. My shoulder bag, which I had with me the night before, was MIA. My eyes bulged with fright. *What the FUCK did I do last night?*

And that's when I faintly remembered stalking back home, marching up tranquil Hill Street between Valencia and Guerrero, shrouded among the shadows of the trees that lined the sidewalks. I remembered feeling very, very angry, stomping on the pavement, flaring my nostrils as if billows of hot smoke were coming out of them, my hands clenched into fists, begging to be put to use. Begging to beat anyone who crossed my path.

My temples felt like they were singed as I lumbered out of bed. I grimaced in pain when I placed my right foot on the floor. The big toe felt bruised, like it had been stubbed repeatedly. I bent over to pick up my Sauconys. The right one was torn where it had covered my toes. *Well that explains the broken drawer*, I thought. Must've kicked the shit out of it.

I picked up the shoes and placed them in my walk-in closet, where I usually tucked them away. I wanted them out of my sight. Didn't want to see them with my sober eyes. Didn't want to be reminded of what I had done.

I limped around the flat to see if I had left my bag elsewhere. While I looked in the kitchen, squinting from the sharp sunlight, I realized that my left arm no longer hurt as intensely as before. I snickered; *how rich is* that, I thought.

Back in my room, I was about to call Tagi. Before I did, I checked my phone for any drunken cellular activity from the night before.

I had made a call to Paola at 1:30 in the morning.

A half-hour-long call.

And I didn't remember one word of it.

Paola answered my first call. After I apologized for calling her late on Friday night, I asked what we talked about.

"You were just really angry," Paola said.

"At you?" I asked.

"No."

"At what—everything?"

"Yeah," she said, pausing. "You kept telling me that you just wanted to kill someone."

"Jesus fucking Christ."

I told Paola what happened that Friday evening. What I *could* remember. (Funny man and truth-speaker Robin Williams—who had been a recovering alcoholic—said this about blackouts: "I believe it's your conscience going into a witness protection program.") But I didn't dare to inquire further about what I had said to her. It was clear that I had gone to some dark, dark place the night before. After we finished talking, I took a shower. With my knees to my chest, I sat in the tub staring blankly at the drain. I allowed the warm shower water to fall onto my shaved head and wash over me, the water pitter-pattering like rain. The morning light and steam encased me like a cocoon. I sat like this for a long time. I was afraid I had done or said something bad to

Tagi. And I could not believe Paola had taken my call the night before, listened to me spew maddened thoughts for *half an hour*. She must *really* care for me, I thought. Why else would she put up with this crazy shit? As I squinted to look through the falling water, I understood that Paola would not forget whatever I had told her during my black-out.

I felt like I was coming undone.

After I called her twice, Tagi called me back. She told me she got ham-mered as well. She met a kind Asian guy who let her crash at his place since there were no more trains to take her back to Oakland after I ditched her. Bless her—she had grabbed my shoulder bag from the club, although my iPod had apparently been stolen at some point during the night. When I asked what happened at the Beauty Bar, why I had left, Tagi said I ran out of the club for no apparent reason. "You were crazy!" she said, without elucidating. And I didn't inquire fur-ther. I told her I was really sorry for leaving her. "I don't know what got into me last night," I said.

My roommate, Amber, stood by the stove in her pajamas. She was shredding cheese over a salad. Amber was beautiful in an earthy way; her brown, wavy hair reached her shoulders. Her face hinted at her mixed Mexican heritage. She was about my age and height. We exchanged good mornings.

"I'm sorry for any ruckus I may have made last night," I said.

"I heard you come in late," Amber said. "You sounded angry. Then you stepped out to the front of the house to talk on your phone."

I snickered.

"Oh yeah, I called Paola at one-thirty in the morning. Real smooth move on my part."

Amber gave a pause.

"I heard you crying outside."

My mouth went agape. Her bedroom faced Dolores Street. The win-dows by her bed hung over the steps that led to our flat.

"I was *crying*?"

"Yeah. A really long time."

"Geez," I said, shaking my head in disbelief. "I *finally* cry about all this, and I can't even remember it. Geez."

I shuffled around Amber to reach into the fridge for my soy milk. I poured myself a bowl of cereal. I didn't have to tell her I got wasted the night before. After living in the bedroom next to mine for two and a half years, Amber knew I was capable of coming home blackout drunk. About a year before, around the time a few of my blood cells must have mutated into cancerous ones, Amber expressed her concern about my heavy drinking. I had come home after a night of binge drinking. She told me she heard me coughing and breathing heavily in my bedroom once I had passed out. She said it sounded bad—like I was choking, struggling to breathe. Amber told me she was worried that one day she would come home and find me dead. She grimaced when she said that, her face full of concern. I told her I knew I had a problem handling my alcohol sometimes. And I appreciated her concern. It took guts for her to say that—that she cared for me as a friend, not just a roommate.

Now when I look back on that drunken episode while undergoing chemo, I can clearly see that it should have been a blaring, five-alarm wake-up call about my drinking. I could have gotten myself in a heap of trouble that night. There is no doubt in my mind that I could have seriously injured someone if they engaged me. And I'm not sure how far I would have gone. Might have kicked someone's head in if given the chance.

I can see now that I was in profound denial of my suffering.

Someday You'll Be Sorry

INT. BALLROOM—NIGHT

Dressed in a black suit and red tie, his head shaved, Juan strides into a ballroom. A thin cloud of smoke wafts in the air from people smoking and dancing. The couples dancing in the middle of the room are elegantly dressed as if they were from the Roaring Twenties. The room is softly lit by crystal chandeliers.

A jazz band plays at one end of the ballroom. The members of the band are dressed in suits with bowties. Sitting behind a celesta, the pianist plays the high, twinkly intro notes to Louis Armstrong's "Someday You'll Be Sorry." Standing front and center beside a vintage microphone, Louis Armstrong blows his trumpet. A bassist, trombonist, clarinetist, and drummer accompany him.

Juan makes his way around the tables. He walks toward the art deco–style bar where several gentleman puff on cigars, their backs against the bar. Leaning his elbow on the bar, Juan faces Mr. Hodgkins, who sits on a stool. He wears a white button-down shirt, black bowtie, and vest beneath his black tuxedo jacket. His derby hat rests on the bar as he stares into his empty martini glass.

JUAN
   Hey there.

Without turning to him, Mr. Hodgkins acknowledges Juan by shifting in his stool. He stares disinterestedly at the top-shelf liquor.

MR. HODGKINS
  Hey.

JUAN
  We'll have a drink later. Let's dance.

MR. HODGKINS
  Must we?

JUAN
  But of course. It's our song.

MR. HODGKINS
  Your song.

JUAN
  No, it's *our* song. If you hadn't come into my life, it wouldn't have
  meant what it does to me now.

*Juan clasps Mr. Hodgkins's shoulder. He leads him past the crowd to
the dance floor. Once they stake a spot, Juan puts an arm around him.
Hip to hip, they dance beneath a chandelier that makes the smoke
around them look like a swirling veil. When Armstrong finishes his
trumpet solo and steps to the microphone, Juan leans his cheek to his
partner's. He softly sings into Mr. Hodgkins's ear while Armstrong
croons.*

JUAN
  "Someday, you'll be sorry. The way you treated me was wrong."

*His eyes watery, Juan caresses Mr. Hodgkins's face. He continues to
sing into his ear, his lips nearly touching Mr. Hodgkins's earlobe.*

JUAN
  "I was the one who taught you all you know."

*They continue to dance to the light tempo while Armstrong gives a
toothy smile to the crowd before he continues to sing.*

JUAN

"There won't be another to treat you like a brother. Someday, you'll be sorry, dear."

The two dance while the trombonist plays a solo. Juan presses his hand to Mr. Hodgkins's face so that they dance cheek to cheek.

JUAN

"There won't be another to treat you like a brother. Someday, you'll be sorry, deeeeeaaaar."

FADE OUT

In the Light

EARLY SUNDAY EVENING, two days after that crazed night out with Tagi, I cycled to the University of San Francisco. Wiping sweat from my brow, I marched to their residence hall where orientation for the writing workshop that I was attending was being held. I felt excited and nervous as I locked Blue to a bike rack in front of the hall beneath an elm tree. It was a gorgeous day. No bleak patches of clouds. No blustery winds to dampen the temperate warmth. Sunlight twinkled through the leaves of the tree that towered above me. For once, it felt like summer in the city.

Inside the residence hall, I grabbed a folder that had my name on it. I walked into the spacious student lounge. It was impossible not to notice how many fellow people of color had gathered for the Voices of Our Nations (VONA) workshops; VONA provides weeklong writing workshops for writers of color taught by writers of color. Paola was the one who encouraged me to apply. (She was taking one of their workshops the following week.) About forty people sat on couches, on love seats, or cross-legged on the carpet of the sunlit room. I took a seat on one of the couches. I wasn't used to this. Growing up in the Bay Area, I had become used to being the minority at all the sexy, cultural-artsy happenings that have nourished me through the years. The art exhibits I visited. The art-house movies I saw. The music shows I caught. The readings I attended. Throughout my adulthood, as I grew more and more racially aware, I began to feel like "the other" in these social situations. Among other Latino Americans, I felt isolated as well—because I read, nurtured my artistic inclinations, and rebelled against being a machista. Looking around the room, overhearing some

101

conversations, I could sense that I was in a room with people who could empathize. I felt giddy.

My body began to cool from the three-mile bicycle ride. I opened my folder to peruse its contents. Inside, I found a name-tag badge to clip to my shirt. In big letters it stated my name and the memoir workshop I was a part of. All around me were Asians, Blacks, people of Middle Eastern descent, and fellow Latinos. Most of them were young, about my age. It was quite different from my Saint Mary's program where I was the only Latino among nearly fifty students (though there were two Latinas in the program). At the far end of the lounge, I saw two familiar faces: Elmaz Abinader, the vibrant, motherly Lebanese American writer who was one of Paola's professors at Mills College; and the one and only Junot Díaz, who won the Pulitzer Prize the year before. They were chatting and laughing it up with a group of students. Meanwhile, many of the other students who walked into the lounge became animated when they met folks in their workshop class. In my memoir workshop alone, I had classmates who came from Brooklyn, Miami, Austin, Los Angeles, and Pittsburgh. The room was charged with infectious excitement.

Soon after, the lounge was packed with over sixty writers and poets. Elmaz and Diem Jones—one of the other VONA cofounders—welcomed us to a roar of applause. Elmaz asked a number of us to part from one side of the room so she could unroll a long piece of butcher paper. Like a red carpet, it ran the length of the sixty-foot-long room. She sprinkled the roll of paper with color markers.

"I want you to write down a few things that you would like to share with everyone," Elmaz said. "Your name. Where you come from. Your nation, or nations. What your ancestors are telling you tonight—and one word to describe how you feel in this moment."

I hesitated at first. There was little space between the folks who knelt over the butcher paper. I was a little shy about potentially bumping tushes with a stranger. Once a teeny space opened up, I crawled and squeezed between two fellow students to grab a marker. I was beaming because it felt like a kindergartenesque activity with grown-up questions to ponder.

After we finished scribbling a little about ourselves, each of us took turns standing up and sharing our responses with the room. For about an hour, the room was filled with bursts of laughter, emphatic sighs, and murmurs as we introduced ourselves. When it was my turn, I told our group that my Spanish-Andean ancestors were telling me to "keep on shining." Our prompts had reminded me of the name my dad wanted to give me, Huascar, which meant "sun of joy" in Quechua. I felt so validated to be a part of that circle. Being in that room with all those fellow writers of color showed me that I was not alone as I had often felt during my adulthood.

The next morning, I cycled through the Mission District, across Market, then zigzagged around the hills in Lower Haight before pedaling up to USF's Lone Mountain campus where our workshops were held. Sweat poured down my face and moistened my bare arms as they glistened beneath the sun. Led Zeppelin's "In the Light" played through my headphones. I had chosen the song on my brand-new iPod, which I typically kept on random play for my crosstown bike rides. Plant was singing a chorus before the song's outro. Page accompanied his vocals with ascending notes on his guitar, bringing the song to a peak as I neared the top of the hill. With not one cloud in the sky, sunlight pouring over me, I closed my eyes. My eyelids became warm blankets of bright orange. I imagined myself grasping that sunlight, imagined it to be like water seeping to my roots, my very core. I imagined myself becoming one with the sun's light (which we are an extension of)—its warmth, its energy healing and nourishing me as I pedaled on.

Gasping for breath, I walked up the steep hill to the campus. My thighs were wobbly while I locked my bicycle to the stair railing of the main building—a towering, prestigious-looking hall. A chipper stream of VONA students strolled by. Wiping my face with a hand towel, I said good morning to Asha, our fiery memoir-workshop teacher from Brooklyn, as she and her daughter walked by. It felt like the first day of school in some beatific universe.

Though our workshop had not even started, I felt triumphant as I walked to our classroom. I didn't scale those hills as fast as I typically would, but I was pleased with my effort. In the face of lymphoma, I had pushed myself. I was not backing down, rolling up in a ball, hiding from the world until I was (hopefully) better. And having lymphoma was not going to keep me from two things I cherished: writing and cycling with the sun shining upon my face.

Jollity with Attali

DR. ATTALI'S ASSISTANT sat on a chair facing me, clipboard and pen in hand. She was beside the door in the small examination room we had congregated to. My legs were crossed while I leaned back to chill in my chair. Wearing a doctor's smock, Attali leaned against the computer desk behind him.

"How was your last infusion?" Dr. Attali asked. He peered at me through his thick-framed glasses. "Still experiencing any arm pain?"

"No more arm pain, thankfully," I said, clasping my hands behind my buzzed head. "I'm feeling great. I've bicycled over twenty-five miles in the past three days."

These oncology appointments were becoming a breeze. Routine. Nothing to worry about. I felt like a patient-ninja in the making. While I sat in the waiting room among the other cancer and HIV patients who came to Ward 86, I forsook the books I usually brought. Instead, I edited the manuscripts for my memoir workshop, which I would cycle back to after my appointment. During our workshop the day before, Asha introduced our group to the six-word memoir. We were given ten minutes to distill our life—who we were—into six words. I was satisfied to have come up with: Desperate to live, hungry for validation.

"Any nausea?" Dr. Attali asked.

"Not really. I barely had to use my nausea medicine after my treatment."

"Any appetite loss?"

"Nope. In fact, I've gained three pounds since my infusion. Right after I did chemo, my hunger went *way* up—like my stomach was screaming, 'Give us some nutrients!'"

They both grinned. His assistant whispered, "That's amazing," as she jotted something down.

"Any night sweats?"

"Nope."

"Fevers?"

"Nope."

"Headaches?"

"Well, I had a headache the other morning when I woke up, but I think it's because I drank too much the night before," I said, flashing a smirk. Attali covered his face with his hand while we filled the room with laughter. I was tickled that I had already managed to joke about that tumultuous night with Tagi.

"Well, you definitely don't want to overdo that," he said in a paternal tone.

"Oh, don't worry. I won't," I said with a tone that bordered on bravado. I must have sounded like a know-it-all. Like I had throughout my adult life, I was so confident I could control my drinking if I simply *willed* it.

After we scheduled my next checkup in a month, I shook hands with Dr. Attali and his assistant. It was the last time I would see him. His oncology fellowship with San Francisco General was ending. He wanted to return to treating patients with melanoma, which was more "challenging" for him.

As I stepped out into the hallway, Dr. Attali gave me a pat on the back.

I felt like such a good boy.

So strong, so in control.

My First Reading

FRIDAY AFTERNOON, AFTER we posed for lots of group pictures and drank some champagne to celebrate the end of our workshop, I said good-bye to my VONA classmates. I walked out of Lone Mountain Main to my bicycle. Situated atop a hill that provided a panoramic view of the surrounding city, I looked out over the concrete jungle—the skyscrapers in the near distance, then toward the Mission, and, finally, to the hospital I had to go to. I changed into my tank top, snapped on my helmet, and blasted Metallica's "Seek and Destroy" from my iPod. For the finishing touch, I put on my aviator glasses. It was "go time"— round two with Mr. Hodgkins. I mounted Blue and pedaled to the parking lot exit. As I zipped down the sharp hill, the air cutting across my face, I let out a loud, "Yeehaw!"

At 4C, I was given a chair next to the big window. Outside, the Bernal Heights hillside spread before me. A few minutes after I arrived, my dad walked into the infusion room.

"Hi, Dad," I said, smiling.

"Hi, son," he said, bending over to kiss my cheek. He was going to drive us to the VONA student reading later that evening. There couldn't have been a more appropriate person. The piece I planned to read was like a dedication to him.

After we chatted for a while, Dad left for the waiting room. I turned to my book and read to pass the time. I was hopeful that the infusion would chug along faster than the first one so we wouldn't miss much of the reading, which was scheduled to begin at six o'clock.

But my second chemotherapy infusion was no wham-bam, come-again-young-cancer-afflicted-man session. Time dragged and dragged with no sign of my chemo fix. By four o'clock, I was muttering "fuck" under my breath whenever I looked up at the clock on the wall. My head began to boil as I sat there bound to the chair, an IV pricked into my arm.

The day before, while sitting at our square circle of desks, I told my VONA workshop class I had lymphoma. I told them I might not be able to make it to the Friday evening student reading since I had an infusion right after our last workshop. "It's going to be my second infusion, so I don't know how my body's gonna handle it," I said, looking around at my classmates, whose expressions changed to sad and serious after the word "cancer" was uttered. "I really, really want to be there to hear everyone read, but I want you to know why I might not be able to make it." By then, I had practice telling a group of people such poopy news. During our last workshop class of the semester, I told my Saint Mary's classmates that I might not be back in the fall since I would still be undergoing chemotherapy.

After I detonated the cancer bomb, I told my VONA peeps that I planned to make something positive of my cancer experience by writing a blunt, this-is-how-it-fucking-is how-to manual for people diagnosed with Hodgkin's lymphoma. A few of them thought it was a great idea. One of my classmates told me how humbled she felt to see me cycle up to the USF campus every morning. I blushed and explained, "I wouldn't want to miss this for anything. Being here, with all of you, has been my happiest week this year." And it was. Asha crooked her head to the side, placed a hand over her heart, then wiped a tear. After class, many of my classmates gave me a big hug along with encouraging words.

Before long, my attending nurse, Vilma, came over to stop my infusion pump from beeping. She was a light-skinned, middle-aged Filipina.

"Can you tell me why it's taking so long for my chemo to get here?" I asked. "I've been here for over *two hours*."

"They have one person working in the pharmacy right now," Vilma said with her Filipina accent. "He's the only person preparing all the medicine for us. Your veins need this saline for the chemo."

If I could have, I would've crossed my arms. Instead, I took a deep breath, hung my head, and sighed. Like a still life, my left forearm lay motionless on the armrest. After the pain I experienced from infusion numero uno, I was afraid of moving that arm whatsoever during treatment.

About a half hour later, my chemotherapy finally arrived. I was ravenous for it. Vilma and Connie—the registered nurse who led the 4C ward—conducted the chemo check. Vilma gave me Ativan and Benadryl pills, then took a seat beside me on a stool.

"I'm going to give you the Adriamycin, bleomycin, and doxorubicin first," Vilma said while unwrapping the syringes. "We'll drip the dacarbazine into your IV. Do you want to increase the infusion flow for it so you can get out faster?"

"Yes, please. I'd really appreciate that."

Minutes later, once the pills kicked in, Vilma connected a syringe to my IV.

"I'm sorry for being a little testy earlier," I said while she pushed the drug into my bloodstream. "I've been attending a writing workshop this week, and we are having a reading tonight. I just don't want to miss it."

"Ah—okay," she said.

Vilma got me out of there as lickety-split as she could. It was 6:45 p.m. when we were done. While she unwrapped the bandage for my IV, I texted Myles—my ridiculously intelligent classmate from Brooklyn—to tell him I was on my way. He was supposed to read a vignette from my memoir piece we had workshopped in case I couldn't drag myself to the reading. Paolita was going to be at the reading as well.

With my dad beside me, I walked into the student lounge. A gauze pad covered the spot where Vilma had infused the Mr. Hodgkins–killin' drugs. (Mr. Hodgkins, *shaking his fist*: "Damn you, Alvarado Valdivia!") The room was packed and abuzz with chatter. I spotted Paola standing beside a refreshment table. We gave each other a hug and kiss before I introduced her to my dad. I beamed as I watched them converse in Spanish.

With no dinner in our tummies, I led my dad on a zigzag path through the crowd to one of the other refreshment tables. We bumped into a few of my classmates and other VONA students I had befriended throughout the week. I was smiley and proud when I introduced them to my pop.

Once the break came to an end, Paola and I sat on the floor near the entrance. A few of the students at the back of the lounge offered my dad their chairs. I was concerned he would feel too far from me in a room full of strangers. I looked back to check on him. Sporting a rare, boyish grin, he nodded and put out his hand, assuring me he was all right.

We clapped, hooted, and cheered on the parade of readers. One by one, they walked to the other end of the lounge to receive a certificate from VONA's director before they read to the crowd. Some read from their spiral notebooks, others from their laptops. A few of the poets paced the floor, staring back at us with intense eyes while they recited their pieces. The lounge was charged with the energy each reader dished.

In good time, my name was called. With page in hand, the room bursting with applause, I turned to Paola and said, "Here I go!" as I stood up. Since I heard about the student reading earlier in the week, I had daydreamt about it a number of times.

The night before, I had trouble falling asleep. In bed, my eyes closed, I imagined myself in front of the crowd. I played out what I would say before I read my piece. I had thought of telling everyone gathered there that I had just come from the hospital, from my second infusion. I imagined how stirring this moment in my life could be. Along with that, I was pumped about reading in front of my dad. When I was twenty-five, still dreaming of becoming an indie filmmaker, he was the one who told me I should be a writer instead. He rarely voiced such opinions, so it made an impression on me. Five years later, my first reading felt like an astounding moment in the making—one that almost seemed to be crafted for a narrative that we simply served—since I was going to read a vignette about my dad *and* have him present to hear it. It was wild and beautiful how all these pieces were aligning.

After I received my certificate, I turned to face the crowd sprinkled throughout the lounge. I took a step forward and set my feet in place.

"Thank you," I said. "This piece is called 'How We Got Our Names, Not Pseudonyms.' All you need to know is that it's about me and my good friend JJ. I want to dedicate this to my dad, who's actually here, sitting in the back."

I lifted my hand and gestured in his direction. Everyone looked over at him.

"Because any good I do, or create, is because of him," I said as the crowd applauded. My father was beaming as he looked around with a buoyant grin.

This is part of what I read:

My full name is Juan Manuel Alvarado Valdivia. My father, to
his credit, did not want to name me after him. He wanted to call

me Huascar. In Quechua, the language the Incans and their Andean descendants presently use, the name means "Sun of Joy." Huascar was the second to last Incan emperor, dethroned by his half-brother, Atahualpa, in a bloody civil war that occurred when the Spanish conquistadors landed on the empire. Huascar, being the last full-blooded Incan emperor, was said to be the favored ruler by the majority of the Incan peasants. It could be that these reasons were why my father wanted to name me after him. My mom talked him out of it since it was an unusual name, even in Peru. Plus, my paternal grandfather was also named Juan, so there was a sexy line of succession to continue. My cousins tell me I should be thankful because a popular juerga, a slang term in my ancestral homeland, is huasca, which means to be shitfaced.

At times, I believe that even though I wasn't named after the second to last Incan emperor, I took and churn within me the spirit that the name would have entailed.

The crowd applauded. I returned to sit beside Paola. She rubbed my leg and smiled. I turned back to my dad. I gave a nod and raised my eyebrows at him. He did the same. It was a gesture I had learned from him as a kid.

The reading stretched on through the night. Though I was captivated by what my fellow VONA peeps were reading and releasing into the world, my eyes became heavy. My head fell forward a few times before I startled awake.

"How are you feeling?" Paola asked at one point, rubbing my thigh.

"I'm feeling okay," I said. "Just really tired."

Before the reading concluded, a few of my classmates and other VONA students walked over to my dad during a break. They shook his hand and chatted him up. All the while, he sat in his chair, smiling and looking up at them as if he were a baby surrounded by cooing adults. Mi papito was like a celebrity! Every time I looked over, he was talking with someone, glowing from the attention.

It'd been a long, long time—years at least, maybe ever—since I'd seen him that happy.

I felt so proud of myself.

111

Frozen Sperm Addendum Number Two

CARMEN, HER BOYFRIEND, Réal, Dad, and I decided to spend our Fourth of July visiting the animal shelter in Fremont. We hoped to find a dog my dad would like. It had been five years since our family dog, Cotton—a short, chubby, poofy-haired American Eskimo—was "put to sleep." My father had wanted a new companion to help fill his lonesome days while my mom worked at the school. Problem was, she didn't want one.

For years, my mother had offered a number of reasons why she didn't want another dog: she didn't want dog hair around the house to sweep up (as if it bordered on a Sisyphean act); she didn't want the overall hassle of taking care of a dog. But my favorite excuse was: "And who's going to take care of the dog while I'm in Peru?"—which only happened once a year for about two months. Our neighbor, Heide, always took care of Cotton on such occasions, just like we always took care of her pets during her vacations. That excuse was also lame since it negated the fact that my dad usually stayed home while she was in Peru. But I also remembered a reason she gave a few months after her father, mi abuelito Grover, died. She had taken care of him in his final months. My mother told me she didn't want another dog just to see it die someday.

After we signed in at the shelter's front desk, we stepped over to a cold, gray hallway lined with doors. It was suffused in sterile white light that reminded me of hospitals. I'd never been to a pound. For years, I was afraid yet curious to visit one. The television images I had seen of shelter dogs locked in their cages, wagging their tails, looking cute and hopeful and desperate at the same time always made me somber.

A cacophony of barks greeted us when we walked into the first kennel block. There were four kennels, which housed an enthusiastic German shepherd mix, a white bulldog with a morose expression and splotches of unhealthy-looking pink skin, and a German shepherd/pit bull mix with spotted fur reminiscent of a hyena (or so Réal and I thought). Carmen came up close to their cages. She knelt to their eye level and said, "Oh, look at you. You're so cute!" My dad stood behind with a faint grin, observing the way they interacted with her. To my surprise—and maybe it was Carmen's infectious gusto—I didn't come close to feeling sad as I watched those poor doggies who wanted nothing more than to not be there. Once I decided that it would be okay to be cutesy yet distant with each of them, I approached their cages. (The last thing I wanted was to give any of them a false sense of hope; that seems like one of the worst things in life.) If they came close to the cage—which most of them did, jumping on it, their paws pressing for contact—I smiled, knelt, and said, "Hey dog! How are you?" I adopted my chipper, child-like, Ralph Wiggum–esque voice to talk to them. "They better be giving you some good food in here!" I would say. Or, "I hope you get out of here, too."

We visited two more kennel blocks. We met a number of adorable, affectionate dogs that deserved love just like any other. As we slowly walked down a fourth kennel block, my mind drifted. I thought about my decision to not freeze my sperm.

"You know, for years I've been hesitant to say that I want my own children," I said to Réal, while we looked at some small mutts. "There are plenty of kids who've already been brought into this world and just need someone to love them. Look at these dogs, man. They're terrific. I think adopting one of them is the *honorable* thing to do, instead of getting a puppy from some pet store."

Réal told me he had said the same thing to Carmen on one occasion. When we left that kennel block, I felt a bit lighter. Relieved. I had no doubts about my decision to forgo sperm storage.

In the end, we walked back to the first kennel block we visited. My dad liked the German shepherd/pit bull mix—the one that reminded me of a hyena. The dog's name was Tanner. The young muscular dog had been dropped off at the shelter by its owner because it was too much to handle. That's what a young, blonde-haired worker told us once we asked if we could take the dog to one of their "get-acquainted areas." She told us that Tanner needed to be walked regularly to get out all the energy he had. Once she said that, Carmen, Réal, and I expressed concern that the dog might be too much for our dad to handle.

The "get-acquainted area" was a fenced-off dirt field sprinkled with shrubs. A horn symphony full of mirth played from a megaphone speaker that pointed toward the field. Tanner tugged brusquely on the leash while we followed the young woman to the gated area. Once inside, she took the leash off. She offered my sister a floppy disc.

"Why don't you go ahead and toss it if you want to play with him," she said. Carmen took it and flicked it about thirty feet. It spun to its descent near the middle of the field. The dog ran after it, getting to the disc moments after it fell to the ground. Tanner snapped it between his jaws in one fluid motion before he turned with his momentum, like a tiny bull charging through a matador's cape. I stood aside. I watched Tanner scamper at my dad, Carmen, Réal, and the shelter employee. He dropped the disc a few feet from them without breaking his stride. Carmen gave a teeny yelp and took a step back when Tanner came jumping at them.

"Come on, Tanner, no jumping," the young woman said. She stepped forward to kneel and grab the dog in order to keep him on the ground.

Dad and Carmen bent down to pet the dog. I could tell they were a bit unsettled. Tanner was turning in semicircles like a dust storm gathering speed. Carmen walked over to the disc and threw it farther. It fell near the end of the fence. The dog chased it down in no time. They stood attentively as Tanner charged back at them, leaping at their thighs.

"He sure does have a lot of energy," Carmen said, trying to pet the dog, who wouldn't stay put.

"He's a ball full of energy, especially when he's let out of his cage," the employee said. "He's not always like this, but he definitely needs *a lot* of exercise. Would you be taking care of him most of the time?"

"No," Carmen said. "He would be staying with my dad."

"Oh, okay."

Réal bent down to pick up the disc. He held it up in the air while Tanner stared at it, his tongue hanging from the side of his mouth. When he flicked it, I looked over at my dad to observe him. Pop was dressed in a sky-blue polo shirt, light khaki pants, and white sneakers that slightly clashed with his clothes. It was an outfit he wore around the house or when we went out to eat—one I expected other old men would wear on cruise ships or in retirement in a place like Florida. With the fence behind him, a golden field in the distance, the horn orchestra playing a triumphant movement, his face contorted into an apprehensive grin as he watched Tanner dart after the disc, I knew he wouldn't adopt the dog. And I could swear that he was, in some form or another, considering his mortality. Or at least I was. I knew my dad was too old, too debilitated from his multiple sclerosis condition to walk a dog like Tanner around the block. A dog like that would yank on the leash and pull my father until he stumbled and fell hard on his face because he wouldn't let go, wouldn't concede. I knew him. I take after him.

Despite the fact that I had been on this planet for thirty years, had understood for quite some time that death is a facet of life, this was the first time I truly understood that my dad would not be around forever. There would be a day when, no matter how many times I would knock on the front door at our home in Fremont, he wouldn't be there to greet me. Gone, absent, like Cotton.

Die, Die My Darling

Or, what I imagined on the bus ride to my third infusion while rocking this song . . .

INT. JUAN'S MEDIASTINUM—DAY

Juan rides a patrol boat up a blood vessel toward his heart. He is dressed in white. Accompanying him are seven mighty lymphocytes who have taken human form. The warriors are cloaked in white robes covered in lymph, which gives them a glowing aura. Their faces are indigenous Andean in appearance: dark-brown complexion, ruddy cheeks, and piercing, slanted brown eyes. They stand like sentinels at the sides of the boat.

The general turns off the boat's engine as they approach the malignant tumor near Juan's heart.

THE GENERAL
　　Quick! Under the tarp!

Juan and his white blood cells slip beneath a tarp that conceals their luminous bodies. Juan and the general peek out at the dark mass ahead.

JUAN
　　Is the amplifier on standby?

THE GENERAL
　　Yes.

The channel darkens as the boat glides into the cancerous mass.

THE GENERAL
Gentlemen, assume your positions.

They stand and toss off the tarp. The white light from their bodies illuminates the dark, fleshy cavern. An army of shadowy figures hovering by its walls coils and hisses at them. The general hits "play" on a boom box connected to two large speakers. The sound of drumsticks clanging together four times in a fast tempo blasts through the speakers. Crashing cymbals and loud hits of the snare drum shake the cavern walls while guitars accompany with thrashing strums. Metallica's rendition of "Die, Die My Darling" fills Mr. Hodgkins's lair. Hundreds of shadowy minions lurking within the caves fly at them from all directions.

Juan and his guardians soar up to face them. The cancerous sycophants are stunned into submission as they meet the sonic waves. They cover their eyes from the light emitting from Juan's guardians.

JUAN
Take that!

Juan kicks one of the woozy shadows blasting through the cavern.

THE GENERAL
¡Muere, muere!

The general wallops the shadowy minions, sending them careening into the cavern walls to wither and dissolve. While the song plays, Juan and his guardians continue to wail on their shadowy adversaries. Mr. Hodgkins's beady, glowing eyes peer out from a cave.

MR. HODGKINS
Get him!

A drove of shadows screech and fly toward Juan. Juan glowers at the horde. He strikes them with a sweeping haymaker. (KAPOW!)

Mr. Hodgkins emerges from the dark. He holds a cane with both hands.

He ascends toward the middle of the cavern. Glowing white, Juan soars up to him. He glares into Mr. Hodgkins's eyes.

JUAN
Looking a little weak these days?

Mr. Hodgkins snarls. Juan can see dark, sagging bags beneath his eyes. Hodgkins looks shell-shocked.

Juan's guardians speed to his side. They shoot beams of light at Mr. Hodgkins as he raises his cane. He winces.

MR. HODGKINS
You—fucks!

Rearing like a cobra, Mr. Hodgkins spits at Juan's head. Juan ducks. The spit falls and sizzles into the blood stream below. Mr. Hodgkins flies back into his lair.

MR. HODGKINS
See you in hell, boy. This is far from over!

FADE OUT

Numero Tres

CHEMOTHERAPY WAS SUPPOSED to be doin' a real number on me by the third infusion. Or so I had anticipated before I began my treatments. A loss of appetite (even for yummy, greasy burritos). Frequent trips to the potty and a subsequent familiarization with every inner crevice of our toilet. Days and nights filled with weary grins. An abundance of inner monologues in which I would stare at the ground and tell myself, *C'mon champ, you can do this.*

But none of that was happening.

The morning after my third infusion—like the first and second time around—I awoke early in the morning with an aching hunger. Having to eat a chocolate-chip granola bar to quench my hunger was far kinder than puking my guts out. And although it was not even an inch long, my cropped hair wasn't falling off in clumps like people shrieking and leaping from a sinking ship.

And so, I was flabbergasted in a mucho-grande-excelente way.

When was this whole battling-cancer deal going to really suck shit?

Since I began my treatment, I had kept a relative leash on myself. Minus VONA week, I refrained from cycling hard. Didn't give myself any challenging writing goals. I was cautious of pushing myself at that critical juncture in my life when I needed to conserve my energy to endure the war being waged within me. But after my third infusion at 4C, I became emboldened. I felt as if I were pirouetting through the summer sky over the city to the string movements that rang electric through my veins. I drew up an ambitious summer reading list. The list was comprised of books that my professors and classmates had recommended to me, or ones I was curious to peruse. I marked their due

121

dates on my 2009 cow-themed calendar. (What can I say; I think they're sacred like any other animal.) Junot Díaz's *The Brief Wondrous Life of Oscar Wao* was due in a few days. *Music Through the Floor: Stories*—by Eric Puchner, one of the visiting professors from the previous semester—was due the following week. Joan Didion's *The Year of Magical Thinking* followed. Then Roberto Bolaño's *The Savage Detectives*, Lorrie Moore's *Birds of America: Stories*, and *You Are Here: A Memoir of Arrival*, the book written by my sweet, charming, and hilarious professor, Wesley, to round it out before classes started in September. To boot, I was invited into the writing group that Paola started with fellow writers of color from Mills College.[*]

From time to time, I would sit at my computer to watch Buster Douglas's knockout of Mike Tyson (again). While I listened to the ringside commentary through my headphones, my mind would flutter with visions of the beauteous, five-mile bicycle ride from the Lafayette BART station to the Saint Mary's campus. I pictured the hills of vibrant green. The trees along the trail. The warm sunlight gleaming on my bronzed arms, nourishing me as I panted and pedaled up the last sharp hill to school. When I imagined myself rolling down the main entrance to campus, sweat streaming down my face, the school's white adobe chapel and its bell tower looming before me, students laughing as they ran on the fields by the entrance, my eyes would well up as I saw myself making it (*I made it!*), chucking my backpack on the vast lawn in front of the chapel, letting Blue fall to the ground while I flopped on my back, arms outstretched, eyes closed, sunlight glittering my eyelids, the most contented smile I had ever felt.

---

[*] Before I was invited into the writing group, Paola and I were wary about having me join due to our relationship. We'd spoken about it before, but I never asked to be a part of the group, though I wanted to join one for some time. After I was introduced, Paola and I agreed that I would be the one to leave if we ever broke up. That seemed fair since she was the one who started it with her chums.

Writing during Wartime

NEAR THE BEGINNING of July, I cycled again to the San Francisco Main Library to read up on all things cancer, such as chemotherapy, lymphoma, even memoirs that others had written about battles with this malady. I had already read Norman Cousins's classic *Anatomy of an Illness*, a book on countering a life-threatening illness with humor and positive inner belief and working with one's doctor to take charge of one's own health. It was time to get further informed. It was also my first attempt at writing a guide on how to survive Cancerlandia. A rather bold prospect on my part, since it was based on the presumptions that (1) I *would not* go belly-up from cancer, and (2) I would manage my personal battle in an exemplary manner worthy of sharing with others. Beneath those fantastic presumptions, though, the desire that gave birth to that idea, the force that drove me to the library that afternoon, the force that has fueled the writing of *this* memoir, was the dire need to create something positive, something beautiful out of this shitty hand I had been dealt.

I stayed at the library a good three hours. The desk I sat at had amassed a pile of books. Among them were *Living with Lymphoma: A Patient's Guide*, *100 Questions & Answers about Cancer Symptoms and Cancer Treatment Side Effects*, *Everyone's Guide to Cancer Survivorship: A Road Map for Better Health*, *The Medical Library Association Guide to Cancer Information: Authoritative, Patient-Friendly Print and Electronic Resources*, and Paul Tsongas's *Heading Home*—a memoir the former U.S. senator wrote about his battle with non-Hodgkin's lymphoma.

The books were loaded with excellent medical information. I skimmed through each table of contents to note what prominent topics were discussed. I turned to the sections that sparked my interest, such as one that discussed how cigarette smoking and alcohol use dramatically increased a person's chances of developing cancer.[*] While I flicked through those books, I jotted down quotes, statistics, and ideas I had about what I could possibly contribute to this discussion. After glancing through the opening pages of Tsongas's memoir, which read like an epistolary novel instead of a dynamic narrative (Tsongas "beat" non-Hodgkin's lymphoma but got it again in 1996; he died shortly after from pneumonia and liver failure at the age of fifty-five—facts that didn't comfort me one bit), I was confident I could write something fresh. Something that could only come from me. Something that could help others.

I left the library with a few books, including *Chemotherapy & Radiation for Dummies*. After I read most of that 380-page book, I created an outline for my how-to guide. The tentative title was *So You Have Hodgkin's Lymphoma: A User's Manual*. (It was a play off of an old book I owned that had what I thought was a hilarious title: *Sex: A User's Guide*.)

Throughout July, I gathered additional research about lymphoma and chemotherapy. I wrote a preface, a four-page, single-spaced section called "Hodgkin's Lymphoma: An Overview with Statistics and Tidbits," and another section titled "How to Tell Your Parents and Loved Ones That You Have Cancer." (In that section, I jokingly advised the reader not to share such bad news when a loved one is operating heavy machinery, such as a car.)

But after that, I couldn't summon the inspiration to write the guide. That advisory section was the last one I wrote. The fall semester was a month away, and I wasn't writing.

I was disappointed in myself. I complained to Paola about my writing woes (though she seemed to be going through her own rut, since she had not written anything since graduating). She told me I was being hard on myself, that I was going through a very difficult situation and shouldn't expect myself to crank out some writing. But I didn't

---

[*] The 2007 edition of *Everyone's Guide to Cancer Survivorship*—a book written by various doctors and medical professionals—stated that there have been about fifty studies that demonstrate that "alcohol consumption has been shown to be a small to modest cancer risk factor, where one drink a day increases the risk 8–10 percent and two drinks a day increases the risk about 25 percent."

want to accept that. I was working a mere fifteen hours per week; I had ample time to generate a consistent output of writing. Having cancer was not an excuse.

One morning, Paola and I walked hand in hand to the 24th and Mission BART station. She was heading to work, while I was going home to get dressed for a short day at the office.

"I'm having a tough time with the guidebook," I said as we stopped at the corner of Valencia and Cesar Chavez—a busy throughway. I stared at the curb, my brow furrowed. "Everything I'm writing has already been written before—and more thoroughly than I could ever write. All I'm doing is condensing the really important information and describing the disease in a more engaging, readable way. But I can't get excited to write it. I don't really have the chance to write in my voice."

The signal turned green.

"You should just write whatever you want," Paola said as we crossed the street. "I'm sure you have a lot you want to say."

Her words were few but magical.

I lifted my head, eyes wide with excitement.

The seed for this memoir was planted.

If Twelve Was Eight

MY FIRST MEETING with Dr. Jaworski—the second in a succession of UCSF fellows who would serve as my oncologists—was perfectly foreboding for my time in his care. I waited two hours to be seen.

When he stepped into the waiting-room doorway, the first thing about Dr. Jaworski that caught my attention was his accent. He sounded German when he called out my name, hesitating before he pronounced my last name. (I would later find out he was from Poland.) He was a white man in his mid-thirties with a medium build and short, dirty-blond hair that was spiky, as though he had just stepped out of the shower. He wore khakis, a button-down shirt, and a tie. I walked out into the hallway, which was bustling with nurses, doctors, and middle-aged patients. Dr. Jaworski shook my hand and introduced himself. He had a warm smile, penetrating blue eyes, and a receding hairline that made his forehead prominent.

"I apologize for the wait," he said in his thick accent, enunciating each word clearly. My green medical file was tucked against his hip. Though I became increasingly upset during the final hour I waited for him, cursing under my breath, sighing with frustration whenever I looked at the time, I grinned and said, "It's cool."

In the examination room, Dr. Jaworski began by asking how I felt. I'd just had my fourth infusion four days before. I told him that my body appeared to be handling the chemo well for the most part. The veins on my left arm were darkening. My forearm had a huge splotch of sickly yellow-greenish bruising. But my hair had not fallen out. I also told him that I wasn't a swirling gust of energy the first three days after my infusions, but it didn't keep me from bicycling for long. I felt strong otherwise. I was willing myself to be. By then, Metallica's "Of Wolf and Man" had become my default fight song. My war call. Before every infusion, the song blared from my headphones as I marched out of the house to the hospital. My spirit roared to the song's nasty staccato riff that sounded like fiery dragon breaths, the thundering snare, the opening verse about a wolf running through the morning mist in search of a fallen lamb. I was the wolf. Mr. Hodgkins was my prey. There was little place in my lymphoma-tinged universe to admit weakness.

Then Dr. Jaworski asked a series of questions that baffled me, although he probably couldn't tell since I didn't furrow my brow or hesitate to answer in a chipper manner. He asked: What cancer do you have? How were you diagnosed? When were you diagnosed? What chemotherapy regimen are you taking? How many infusions have you undergone? How many cycles of treatment did Dr. Attali recommend?

It was puzzling because I presumed that Dr. Attali would have provided him with a summary note, a CliffsNotes version of each of his patients. I figured Dr. Jaworski's job, his homework, was *to know* these elementary facts about my prognosis. But he was new, and there was too much I didn't know about his line of work, so I didn't want to immediately presume he was incompetent. Instead, I figured those questions were a pop quiz of sorts—a test that would allow him to size up his new patients. To see how informed I was about my disease and treatment. To see how much fight I had in me. Throughout our Q&A session, Dr. Jaworski sat straight in a chair opposite me, his legs crossed, my medical file open on his lap. He was attentive, but now I was left with the impression that he was overwhelmed—like a student who had not studied hard for a test.

Although we had just met, and although I had yet to undergo a CT scan during chemotherapy to see if the treatment was working, Dr. Jaworski told me something that filled me with excitement: he was leaning toward doing the minimum of four cycles of ABVD. Eight chemo infusions. He was concerned about the risks involved with prolonged chemotherapy.

Despite the fact that Dr. Attali seemed to have his shit together more than Jaworski—more assured, more in control, like a veteran physician—and even though he told me we would likely complete at least five cycles of treatment, I was all too eager to embrace Jaworski's recommendation. Less chemo seemed like a terrific idea! His logic for it seemed sound. If I had to undergo four cycles of treatment, I would only have two infusions during the fall semester. Hot damn, I was potentially halfway done!

My next appointment with Dr. Jaworski was scheduled for four weeks. We would discuss the results of my CT scan, which had already been scheduled for the following day. Although I felt optimistic that the chemotherapy was doing its destructive work (like a napalm shower of my body if it were a city occupied by hostile invaders), I was worried about the results. It was a gnawing, indomitable sense of worry that no words could sweep out of my mind.

What if the treatment wasn't working?

What then?

I slept poorly that night. Four or five hours at most. Two swigs of vodka were needed to lull me to sleep.

I fell asleep during the half-hour-long CT scan the next morning. My arms were stretched out above my head as if I were Superman, flying back and forth through that whirly-sounding machine, up, up, and away.

Crows

A FEW DAYS later, I had another rough night of unsleep. At around three in the morning, I made the mistake of looking at the time on my VCR, which only made me feel more frustrated. Groggy, I remained in bed, thinking that descent into sleep was a matter of breaths away.

Then I heard a crow caw nearby. It sounded like it was perched in one of the trees in our backyard. *How unusual*, I thought. I have *never* heard a crow at night, let alone in the thick of a city. Then it cawed again. My eyes shot open. The caw sounded like it came from a different location. As if the crow were circling above the house. With my heart thumping, I stared at the dim ceiling, waiting, waiting to hear it again. I could feel my eyes bulge when I thought I had heard the faint flapping of its wings passing above.

Many years before, my family would periodically gather to watch Gregory Nava's *My Family*, starring Edward James Olmos, Jimmy Smits, and Jennifer Lopez (when she used to look more Latina!). The film, which chronicled the history of a Mexican American family that settled in East Los Angeles, was like lore for nuestra familia. We watched it a handful of times. (I always identified with Jimmy—the "family fuckup." The one who carried all the rage and injustice for the Sanchez family.) There is a scene in the film where one of the Sanchez kids, Chucho, evades death by being pulled out of a turbulent river as a helpless infant. Once he grows up to be a mota-dealing vato in East L.A., he is shot down by the police for killing a rival gangster. Olmos's narrator tells the audience that it was "the spirit of the river" taking Chucho's life after all those borrowed years. For years, I incorrectly remembered a crow—instead of a white owl—looking down on Chucho when he is running from the police on the night he dies: an omen of his death.

And so, years later, on that sleepless night while I lay in my bed with a cancerous tumor in my chest, I became scared of crows. I was afraid one was circling. Waiting to take me.

Would You Like Some Hair with Your Cereal?

SUNDAY MORNING, AUGUST 2, I sat at our kitchen table. I was chillin' in my pj's and slippers. Soft sunlight fell on the bowl of Honey Bunches of Oats before me. The house was quiet. Outside our window, the sky was a cozy gray, enveloping the neighborhood in a soft mist. It was a week after my fourth infusion.

Though I had always anticipated it, it was nonetheless peculiar when I flicked my fingers through my cropped hair and saw a few hairs fall into my cereal. They seemed to tranquilly float in the milk. I ran my hand through my hair again. Like a magic trick, a few more hairs floated down into the bowl, dotting the milky liquid canvas. *Oh*, I thought, *this must be the chemo*. Or maybe it was because of the drags I pulled from a joint the night before at an artsy party?

Years and years before, when I was a pimple-ridden teenager, I once pulled out twenty or thirty of my black locks as I read a book in bed. I did it more out of boredom and fascination for the hair follicles I could pull out without pain. I placed them in a little pile over my white pillow. Pulling them out had taken some effort—minutes of grabbing and yanking my hair.

Now my hair was falling out by merely skimming my hand over my head.

By then, nine weeks into treatment, I had begun to believe that I might be part of the exceptional 5 percent of patients who do not experience hair loss from chemotherapy. But those fallen hairs showed that something unnatural, something very wrong was happening inside my body.

My tranquil Sunday morning breakfast was kaput. And just like that, the gray sky outside felt ominous and dreary.

The Judas Kiss

I PLAYED THIS ferocious, thundering Metallica song again and again while I cycled down the hills of Moraga. Or along the city's streets. Sometimes I would imagine myself dressed in black—like death incarnate—barreling toward Mr. Hodgkins on a motorcycle armed with machine guns on its handles (quite unimaginatively like the Batpod). The lights from the skyscrapers blur past me like flares shooting through the dark sky. Mr. Hodgkins is standing in a vacant parking lot. His cackles echo off the buildings surrounding him. *That's it, come get me!* he says. His laughter infuriates me further. It feels like there is a bonfire raging in my chest.

My foot presses down hard on the pedal as I round a corner onto the street that leads to him. The motor roars as I slice between traffic, my hands gripped tight on the handles. The speedometer needle spikes. Eighty, ninety, one hundred miles per hour—the wind, the night howling in my ears. I couldn't care less if he is standing next to a building. Couldn't care less how much it would hurt to run full speed into him, into a wall.

You shouldn't have fucked with me, I say, my eyes fixed on Mr. Hodgkins as I accelerate toward him, my pupils opening like pools of black.

After I run him down, his derby hat flipping high up into the air while I bounce off the brick wall that the motorcycle crumples into, I pounce on him and pound his skull, fist to face, fist to face, his dark blood splattering over my knuckles, pouring out of his mouth and nose before I tear off his bloodied face, chomp by chomp, chunk by chunk, until he is a faceless pulp bludgeoned into the pavement, a mangled corpse that I stand and lean over while I scream and scream and scream until the concrete around him splinters like broken glass.

Paola's Twenty-Eighth Birthday

WITH HER HEELS clicking on the sidewalk, Paola and I left her office walking hand in hand amid the flock of office workers heading back home for the day. It was a beautiful summer day in early August—her twenty-eighth birthday. The sun gleamed off the skyscrapers. A cool zephyr blew. Although she suggested we take the streetcar, we walked to the Gordon Biersch Brewery Restaurant since I thought it wasn't too far away. It turned out to be nearly a mile away, though the view of the sparkling bay and Bay Bridge while walking near the Embarcadero was awe-inspiring. (I did feel bad that she had to walk so far in her heels). While I stared up at the bridge, Paola's hand in mine, I had a fleeting thought—that sometime in the not-so-distant future we might not have the opportunity to easily see this bridge. After her graduation, Paola told me she hoped to move back to Seattle to be close to her family. Carmen had lived there a few years. I visited her once. It was a beautiful, laid-back city—a place I could see myself moving to with Paolita if all turned out super-duper well between us. That day, I had reason to be hopeful. When Paola showed me around her office, her colleagues smiled and shook my hand and said, "It's nice to meet you," as though they had heard pleasant things about me.

The only folks who joined us for happy hour at Gordon Biersch were my old friend Sunil and his wife. We attended junior high and high school together in Fremont. We were jesters in spirit. The class clowns. Senior year, he was voted "Most Likely to Star in a Movie with Chris Farley," while I was voted "Most Likely to Be Found Watching *Scooby Doo* and Eating Lucky Charms (Kid at Heart)." The last time we'd seen each other was five years before, when we worked in the South Bay.

Though we never spoke about my disease, Sunil must have seen my recent cancer-related posts on his Facebook feed. Must have figured it was as good a time as any to catch up with me.

Once darkness fell over the city, Sunil and his wife dropped us off at the Cat Club for a night of dancing to eighties music. By then, only nine o'clock, I was already drunk.

The rest of that Thursday night—however long it was—is a faint blur. Like a pitch-dark void. When I have tried to recall that night—which is like a dread-leaden nightmare to me now—all I can conjure are some fleeting moments: meeting Apollo (a.k.a. the Greek), a kind, demure, clean-cut writer who went to grad school with Paola, and seeing my homeboy Scott, who I hardly knew back then. (I have exclusively relied on his memory of that night to reimagine it.) The one vivid recollection I have from that night is standing with my back against the bar closest to the club's entrance. I was smacking Scott's back, congratulating him for getting married to his longtime girlfriend. Scott's beefy white half-brother was in town to attend their civil ceremony. *All right, let's do some shots!* I roared. The three of us downed celebratory tequila shots. End of memory. What I *don't* remember is slamming down my shot glass, stretching my arms out along the crowded bar counter, and rearing my head to let out a wooooooo-howl (as Scott puts it). The people standing around us stared at me. They appeared bemused. Scott and his half-brother certainly were. (It's worth mentioning that Scott has a talent, a propensity, for attracting crazy people.) Then we downed another shot.

The night raged on. I can't recall one song that was played. Nor do I remember dancing with Paola's party—her three roommates and about twelve friends and former classmates—in the main dance room. And I certainly don't remember tossing my drink over the head of one of Paola's roommates while we danced beneath the flashing lights. I'm not sure why I threw my plastic cup. (I did not necessarily dig this particular roommate, but I wouldn't say I *disliked* her.) I also don't remember being subsequently shown the door by Paola with Scott's help. Before Paola nudged me out of the club, she had told him, "We gotta get him out of here."

Outside, Paola and Scott leaned me against the building. Paola's friend Fabian was in tow. I began to slump against the wall, my head tilted back, eyes all wobbly like I'd just been walloped. A few feet from us was a street-cart vendor grilling onions and hot dogs. Next door was another club. A few people took drags from their cigarettes on the sidewalk. Others thumbed away on their phones. Then I started screaming, "FUCK YOU MOTHERFUCKERS! I HAVE CANCER!"

Scott, a stocky, bespectacled, over-six-foot-tall Mexican American with a scruffy face and moustache stood beside me. He was prepared to lock his arms around me. Paola and Fabian stood nearby on full alert.

I continued to scream, to no one, to everyone, "FUCK YOU! I HAVE CANCER!"

About six feet away, near the corner of 8th and Folsom, a young hipster couple stared at us. They stood close together, arms around each other. He was smiling while his girlfriend giggled.

"What are ya looking at, you white bitch?" I shouted. I was *wasted* to have said shit like that.

They must have surmised that I was just some drunk motherfucker because they didn't say anything back. The lanky boyfriend kept his back to me while she peered over his shoulder.

"Fuck you. . . . I have cancer," I slurred. "I'm gonna die! I'M GONNA FUCKING DIE!"

Paola talked to Scott and Fabian about getting me into a cab. That's when I bent over like I was ducking a clothesline and tore off down the sidewalk, past the hot dog vendor. I didn't stagger-run too far since I was drunk. And being the crazy fuck that he is, Scott howled at my sudden transformation from zombie-drunk to loco-on-the-run. Paola and Fabian walked over to me. When they approached, I ran again to evade them. The Cat Club bouncer told them I couldn't be in front of the club in my state. I dashed away from Paola a few times before I willingly went back to them, muttering something to the effect of, "All right, all right, all right."

Scott and Fabian stood beside me as I leaned against a building next to the Cat Club. My head was bent forward and my eyes were closed as though I had passed out standing. I squinted and peeked out of the corner of my eye at the hipster couple. The young woman continued to look over at us.

"The fuck you looking at?" I slurred.

Scott put his arm around my back.

"Come on, man, it's all right," he said with his faint Texas drawl.

139

"Let's get you something to eat."

Together, we stepped over to the hot-dog vendor. A pile of onions and a row of steaming sausages sizzled on the grill. A few revelers stood beside the short Mexican vendor and his pushcart, devouring their hot dogs.

Scott bought me a hot dog while Paola turned back and forth, from keeping an eye on me to looking out for a cab. Fabian was out on the street, trying to flag one down to haul me off. Typically I cherish these street vendors, most of whom set up near popular bars in the Mission on weekend nights. But I suddenly started insulting the poor guy in Spanish, *while I ate* the hot dog he had just grilled for me. A new low in my life. The man looked off with an indifferent gaze—collateral damage for the population he serves. Scott put his arm around my back to drag me away.

Fabian and Paola managed to flag down a cab. The cab driver stopped in front of the club. Paola scurried over to him. "Can you take us to 22nd and Dolores?" she asked. When she turned around to lead me into the cab, I tore off down the sidewalk again. The cab driver was no fool. He bailed.

Paola, Scott, and Fabian kept watchful eyes on me after they coaxed me back near the club. Leaning against the wall again, I proceeded to dramatically sag to the side. That's when I noticed a group of hulking motorcyclists clad in black leather down the street. Earlier that night, Scott had seen one of them making out with one of the male bartenders. Apparently I had too.

"Fucking white faggots!" I screamed.

They hollered back.

Then three of them stomped in our direction.

When they were halfway down the shadowy street, the six motorcyclists appeared small—at least to Scott. But as they approached, he could see that they were *huge*. Built like sequoias. Bald, pierced, with thick body-builder necks. They were taller than Scott. And they had spikes on their leather jackets.

"Hey, what's this guy's fucking problem?" one of them asked as the group marched up to us.

Having grown up in a family and Texas town full of rednecks, Scott—a self-professed "half-Mexican, half-redneck"—quickly surmised the peril I had placed us in.

"We love you white people," Scott said in a jokey, please-don't-beat-the-living-crap-out-of-us tone. He stood between me and the leather-clad hulks. My head was lolling to the side. "I'm sorry. My buddy's had too much to drink."

"Then what the fuck's wrong with your friend?"

"He's drunk."

"Well get him the fuck outta here!"

Paola flagged down a taxi. Like a Pavlovian cue, I lumbered down the sidewalk yet again.

Two of the bikers ran after me. Scott trailed behind. One of the bikers corralled me by the neck while the other helped to shove me into the cab. Paola slid in beside me. Before the cab drove off, she looked back at Fabian and Scott with an embarrassed, worried expression. She had me dropped off at my home.

Paola posts a generous number of pictures on her Facebook profile. She posts photo albums for nearly any special occasion: Halloween, her graduation, you name it. She would post them in their own respective albums. But there was one glaring exception: she never posted any photos from her twenty-eighth birthday.

At some point in the night, I had mustered enough presence of mind (*presence of mind—ha!*) to set my cell phone alarm for my infusion the following morning.

Chemo—Hung-the-Fuck-Over

IN RETROSPECT, I suppose this says a lot about me then, but before I began chemotherapy, I thought, *It wouldn't be a good idea to do this hungover.*

Boy, was I fucking right.

Friday morning, I awoke in a state of painful bewilderment from the alarm that startled me. My temples throbbed as I crawled out of bed to reach my phone, which I had left—as I always did when the alarm was set—a few feet away on the floor. Hanging halfway out of my bed, I probably didn't look altogether different from Mike Tyson did when he got knocked out in Tokyo: googly-eyed, crawling on the canvas, desperately reaching for his mouthpiece.

Oh shit, I have to get ready for chemo.

How did I get here?

Oh god, oh god, oh god, oh god—what the FUCK did I do last night?

Before I dragged myself into the shower, I noticed that my shoulder bag was not resting beside my dresser. Also missing in action was the jacket that Paola had given me for my birthday. The makings for a long, agonizing day were already set.

And both of my parents would be at the infusion.

Since my mom was back in the country, she wanted to be at the hospital for my fifth infusion. She and Dad had asked if they could pick me up that morning to take me to the hospital. Thank god I had agreed. A bus ride on the crowded 48 to the hospital would have been abominable in my hungover state. I might have puked along the bumpy ride.

143

In the infusion room, I was seated in one of the chairs facing the front doors. Not only were my parents standing by the doorway, looking over me, but anyone could have peered in to see me, hanging my head from pain. From shame. Once I sat down, I promptly took off my shoes, reclined the chair, and accepted a blanket from Vilma. This was uncharacteristic of me. I usually sat in my chair for the first hour or two, reading, eating my apple and banana while sipping some water. I placed my left arm on the armrest like an offering, as if it were my burden. I turned away from my parents. Tried to hide my face from their sight. The red eyes. The bags beneath them—the incriminating evidence. On top of my sour gut, I had this sick, sick feeling that I had done something horrible the night before.

If being hung-the-fuck-over during chemo wasn't bad enough, the veins on my left arm had decided to revolt. They were tight like cords, but I didn't run my finger over them for fear that it would hurt. They were tired, tired, tired of intruders! Vilma sat on a stool beside me and poked a needle into three spots on my forearm without finding a vein that would take an IV. Getting that needle in place was always the most nerve-racking part of the entire infusion. By the time she pricked into a vein by my wrist, which hurt because it felt like it was poking against bone, I wanted to wail in a disgusting display of self-pity. For the pain my dumbfuck ass had brought on itself. For being so fucking stupid to have drunk so much, *yet again*. For fucking up, yet again—in all likelihood—a relationship, a good thing in my life.

Between fleeting sleep and dejecting wakefulness, I squinted when I glanced around the room. The lights seemed hideously bright. I caught glimpses of my mom and dad as they stood against the wall with blank, worried faces. I peered over at Vilma, her glasses on, a medical mask covering her nose and mouth while she hovered over my arm to inject a syringe full of chemo into my IV. I couldn't look my parents in the eye. I shut my eyes. I prayed for sleep, where this nightmare could temporarily cease.

Later that afternoon, my parents and I arrived at our home in Fremont. The bony top of my hand was wrapped with a bandage. I slept most of the day, cuddling next to Negrita.

Earlier, I had called and texted Paola. She had not responded. I implored her to tell me what had happened the night before. She eventually called and reluctantly told me that I had lost control of myself. Went crazy. Had to leave the club after I became "really aggressive" on the dance floor. She told me I had to be taken away in a cab.

When I persisted in asking exactly *what* I had done, Paola told me she did not want to talk about it. And that's when I dropped my questions, hung my head, and apologized further.

Paz

AFTER DINNER AND chai at a popular Indian restaurant on trendy Valencia Street (a.k.a. Hipsterlandia), my friend Jonathan (a.k.a. Jonny, or Jonnycito) and I hurried over to the San Francisco Buddhist Center a few blocks away. I had suggested that we check out their drop-in beginner's meditation class. As my treatment progressed, I was experiencing more and more insomnia, although Dr. Attali had told me it shouldn't be a side effect from the chemo. But two nights before, like many before it, I lay in bed, my mind seemingly incapable of taking that turn, clicking into place, in order to ease into sleep. I thought meditation could help to calm my mind. For years I had flirted with the notion of practicing meditation. After I became an atheist when I was nineteen, Buddhism was the only religion that somewhat appealed to me.

Jonny is one of the people who was really there for me after I was diagnosed with lymphoma. He is a testicular-cancer survivor who was once given a 50/50 prognosis of survival. Though we had never been super close over the ten years we had known each other since meeting in a humanities class, I always considered him a dear friend. Jonny has always been slight in build and light in complexion, with short brown hair that is combed in a manner that any mother could be proud of. He's seven years older than I am. Like me, he looks youthful for his age. When he smiles, his front teeth protrude slightly. It gives him a disarming charm. It would be an understatement to say that he's soft and tender in voice, to the point where I simply cannot imagine him *ever* raising his voice at anyone (though he does sport a hearty laugh). In a metropolis boasting a 15 percent gay population, Jonny is one of the few gay men I have met who has remained a friend after finding out that I'm straight. He is one of those rare spirits—like a walking bundle of sunlight—that any of us would be fortunate to ever have in our lives.

Years ago, Jonnycito sent me a heartbreaking e-mail in which he told me he had HIV. It was a secret he held from nearly everyone—including his family—for years. When he got diagnosed with testicular cancer shortly afterward, he quit his job and moved back home with his parents. Once he fully recovered from his cancer battle, Jonny moved back to San Francisco—a few months before I was diagnosed. He volunteered for the STOP AIDS Project as well as the public clinic where I saw my doctor. He was a volunteer counselor at their HIV clinic where I got tested after my trip to Thailand. I was tremendously proud of him, proud of all the effort he was putting into helping others. Conversely, he was proud of me for continuing to work and go to school. He didn't know how I could do it. When he told me this, it was the only time I wondered how I did it.

The Buddhist center was located in a nondescript building across the street from a parking garage. It was boxed between a hardware store with scratched windows and a gray warehouse that served more as a canvas for graffiti. In the back of the main room, a group of ten people—mostly our age or a bit younger—sat on cushy couches. A bespectacled, slender white man in his mid-fifties with a shaved head sat on one end of a couch. He sat with impeccable posture. With his hands in his lap, he faintly grinned at whoever was introducing themselves to the group. He spoke with a soft voice with a British accent. Once Jonny and I introduced ourselves, we all walked into the shrine room.

The room reminded me of a bomb shelter with its thick brick walls. A semicircle of mats faced a golden Buddha statue. Jonny and I took neighboring mats. The Buddhist leader and his young male assistant took their spots, flanking the statue that gleamed beneath a small light that beamed down on it. We sat cross-legged with erect postures on cushioned pillows. We draped our lower halves with thick burgundy blankets like the group leader had done.

The leader guided us into closing our eyes. My hands rested over my knees, palms open. The room was quiet other than his proper, British voice. He guided our attention to our shoulders, then down to our lower back, legs, and feet entwined beneath us. Once we settled into our postures, the silence of our thoughts, he guided us into the meditation practice of *metta bhavana*—the cultivation of loving-kindness.

148

First, he asked us to think of someone we saw on a daily basis but never spoke to. A coworker or, say, the lobby attendant of the building we worked at. He asked us to think of them, to send compassion, love, and wishes of peace to them. A bell chime rang, echoing through the room. Then, he instructed us to do the same for a good friend. I directed my loving thoughts to Jonny, who sat a few feet away. The bell rang again. The leader asked us to direct our loving intentions to someone we were in conflict with.

My right foot began to throb with discomfort by the time we got to the last prompt. I could feel my pulse slow while I concentrated on inhaling and exhaling the finite breath within me. Though no one in that room could see—unless they were cheating and not keeping their eyes closed—my lips were contorted into a faint grin. Call me a hippie, but I felt my heart basking from the love I had sent out, the gratitude I had for the breaths I could take at that moment.

"Now I want you to think about yourself," the leader said. He paused for a long time. The room was still, absent of the city's ceaseless murmur. "Listen to your heart beat. You deserve love. You deserve peace."

When he said those final words, I muffled a gasp that shook through me. "You deserve peace" felt like a punch to my stomach. I could feel my eyes welling up. Had I not been a part of a meditation class that was supposed to be silent, I could have filled that room with my sobs. Those three words coursed deep within my heart. I had not done enough throughout my life to give myself peace.

Momma's Birthday

PAOLITA AND I drove to Fremont on Saturday, August 15, for a double-whammy celebration: my mom's fifty-fourth birthday and the anniversary of Arequipa's founding. My parents were having a barbecue. It was the first time Paola met Mariana, Rick, and my uncle José Luis. She would also meet Tagi for the first time, since she happened to be visiting a family friend that afternoon in Union City, the equally forgettable town north of Fremont. (Paola knew that Tagi and I had a drunken one-night stand years ago when we were both in relationships.) I was super curious to see what Tagi would think of her. In the five years we had been friends, Tagi was one of the few people who had met most of the young women I had dated. She was also one of the few people who I talked to about love, about my relationships. In that regard, she was my closest confidante.

We stood and drank cuba libres and Coronas by a semicircle of fold-out chairs on the back lawn with Mariana, a sloppy-drunk Rick, and two of my mom's girlfriends. I nursed my drink. I was afraid of getting too drunk in front of Paola. When I greeted my mom's friends, they asked, "How are you doing?" I had become accustomed to such queries from everyone. It made me feel like a walking health report. In short time, I had developed a default response whose wording I tweaked for whoever asked. As always, I gave them positive reports, told them I had gained weight—five pounds—since I began treatment. I told them I still cycled around the city, even jogged around the neighborhood from time to time. They grinned and said, "It's good to see that you're handling it so well." I shook my head and chuckled, then gave a cryptic response that only Paola—who stood beside me—understood:

"Well, I am, for the most part. But there've been times when I haven't handled it so well."

Once the anticuchos (marinated beef hearts), juicy steaks, and corn were grilled, we gathered at the tables beneath our patio roof. I sat at the head of a picnic table, my father on the opposite end. He was flanked by my mom and her brother, Tío José Luis. Eight of us sat at that table while Mariana, Rick, Heide, and my cousin Juan Luis sat at a table beside us. Paola sat to my right, facing Carmen, who had driven up from Los Angeles that day. They exchanged pleasantries, a few easy questions like, "How was your trip?" Conversation at our table was humdrum. It felt like the makings of a long afternoon. Then Tagi called.

I stepped away from the table to take her call. She had gotten lost after she stopped at a Safeway to buy flowers for my mom. Once I figured out where she was in Fremont, I gave her directions to our house. I was tickled that she was going to meet my family.

A few minutes later, Tagi showed up at the front door holding a splendiferous bouquet of flowers. As always, she was warm and smiley and excitable. I led her out to the backyard. Both tables greeted her with gusto.

"Mom, this is my good friend Tagi. Tagi, this is my mom," I said, standing beside my friend, proud to introduce them.

"Happy birthday! I've heard so much about you!" Tagi said. She held the bouquet out to her before they exchanged a big hug and kisses on the cheek.

"Oh, thank you!" my mom said in her accented English. She put the flowers to her nose and took a whiff.

"They're beautiful. Oh, you shouldn't have," Mom said with a playful wag of her hand.

"But it's your birthday!" Tagi said.

I was beaming.

Carmen scooted over so Tagi could sit beside me. For the next two hours, our table was charged with the energy she brought. She engaged my parents, sisters, Paola, and me with thoughtful questions. The two of us laughed as I cracked jokes about cancer. When Tagi left, she took the excitement with her.

For the rest of our drawn-out barbecue (which included a toast to Arequipa's founding by the Spaniards and my mother blowing out the candles on her cake), Paola sat beside me and said very, very little. With her friends she was a gabbing machine to the point of sometimes being annoying, since her voice had a nasally quality when it was raised. I quietly asked her, at least two or three times, "Are you bored?" Each time, she shook her head with a faint grin and continued to sit straight. At one point I said to Paola, "You know, you don't have to stay if you don't want to. You came all the way out here to celebrate my mom's birthday. You've already done some good work tonight!" But she continued to sit there and not say a word. Observing but not engaging.

Paola left well into the night. My mom was especially pleased she had visited. Earlier that evening, before it became dark, Mom brought out the binder where she kept my old report cards and all of the birthday cards I had ever given to her. (She kept a binder for each of us kids.) Sitting side by side in the living room, she flipped through it with Paola. Paolita saw birthday cards I had drawn with crayons when I was a wee one. It was evident that my mom liked her. Paola was a polite, sharp-dressing working professional with no tattoos or facial piercings, a Latina who spoke fluent Spanish. How could my mom *not* love her?

I walked Paola to her car. We hugged and kissed as I thanked her for coming out. It meant a lot to me. Most of my relationships did not last long enough to bring a girlfriend home to meet my parents. By then, I began to believe I might have finally found the love of my life in Paola. Three days after her horrendous twenty-eighth birthday, Paolita drove us to Baker Beach in her sporty Mazda. That sunny afternoon, the Golden Gate Bridge looming to our right, the lush green Marin hillside across the sparkling bay, I felt a sense of peace as I sat beside Paola, eating the burritos we had brought. I felt like a mangy mutt that had been picked from the pound and given another chance to prove it could be a good companion. Perhaps I had found someone who believed in me so much that she was willing to overlook those mad, drunken incidents she witnessed in our short time together. The kind of eruptions that helped scare a few women away.

Once I walked back to the front door of my parents' home, I felt a mix of emotions. I hung my head pensively. I felt bad that Paolita had stayed as long as she did. She must have been bored. I felt I was to blame. But most of all, I felt bummed that she didn't have a good time with us. At least that's why I *thought* I felt disappointed in that moment.

But months later, I would figure out why I felt so disappointed.

Pismo

RIGHT AFTER MY sixth infusion, Paola and I hit the road for a weekend in Pismo Beach, a three-and-a-half-hour drive south. The getaway was planned for the week before my fall semester began. With my head resting against the window, I slept most of the way there.

When I awoke from my Ativan-Benadryl stupor, Paola jazzed up the ride with tunes from her iPod shuffle. Her playlist was mostly Spanish-language fare that belied her Mexican upbringing, clásicos like Banda el Recodo and Vicente Fernández. She spiced it up with some modern goodies like my girl Julieta Venegas and a band named Belanova. She played their song "One, Two, Three, Go!" It was a ridiculously catchy pop song that made me bob my head. Listening to it, my mind raced away in daydreams of running and soaring through the sky, weaving through highway traffic as if I were Sonic the Hedgehog with a jet pack. Paola noted how excited I got about their song. She kept the Belanova goodness going with some of their chill yet danceable songs.

Then Pismo Beach was in sight. To the right of the highway, the Pacific Ocean spread before us.

Back in my early twenties, I used to drive past Pismo Beach to visit Carmen in Santa Barbara. After high school, she left to study at UC Santa Barbara. I would always slow down when I saw the beach—the blue ocean stretching beyond it, glistening beneath the sun. I always cruised past the beach with longing eyes, as if it held a mysterious promise.

On one of those drives back home to Fremont, I decided to check it out. I still felt melancholy from a relationship that had come to its end. All I wanted was to walk on the beach, to hear the lapping waves, to feel the ocean breeze. I was curious to know if it was as serene as it appeared from the highway.

I drove to the main pier. With my camera bag slung over my shoulder and my tape recorder in my pocket, I walked past some young, raggedy skater hippies who sat on the sidewalk watching their friends attempt kick flips in the parking lot. The beach area beside the pier was practically vacant. I had the beach to myself.

I kicked off my flip-flops and walked out toward the waves. The sun was setting over the Pacific, painting the sky in swirls of purple and pink. I took out my film camera. Squinting through its lens, I set the best composition and snapped a picture to document the moment. With the sand sifting between my toes, I walked out close to the waves. I hit the "record" button on my tape recorder, said "Pismo" into the microphone. I recorded the lapping waves for half a minute before I left.

It was bittersweet to be there without anyone to share that sunset with. Although I was tempted to walk around the small beach town to buy some food for the road, I decided not to. I promised myself I would only stop in Pismo Beach again with someone I loved.

And I kept that vow.

Five years later, I rode beside Paola as she drove us into town.

Somewhere in my heart, I hold treasured memories from that weekend. Like falling asleep with Paolita, cuddled on the couch while we watched the copy of *Amelie* I brought. Brushing our teeth together in the bathroom. Making sweet love. Sleeping in. Waking up next to each other the following morning. Spending the afternoon at the beach atop our blanket, a cold, gray cover of clouds above us while I trudged through the last half of Bolaño's *The Savage Detectives* and Paolita read Ana Castillo's *The Guardians*. Once a light rain chased us from the beach, we hung out in the hotel's pool during the evening. We smiled at each other to the pitter-patter of raindrops on the pool's surface.

Before we left town on Sunday afternoon, Paola and I drove to downtown Pismo Beach. After an hour of reading at the beach, we walked to Splash Café. It was the restaurant my roomie, Amber, had recommended; she grew up in a neighboring town and told me they made the best clam chowder she has ever had. And we were hungry with a capital H. We excitedly placed our order. After we handed them our cash, I pogo-hopped along the counter, then wormed through the crowded café. We took a table near the back entrance. Paola told me she was going to walk to the car to get her big bottle of water. I volunteered to fetch it.

The sidewalk bustled with people clad in sunglasses and sandals. The sun had finally emerged, though the temperature was still San Francisco–like in the low sixties. Before I made it to the first street corner, I felt a coughing fit come over me. It was the dry cough I had developed in the past few weeks—one that only happened when my tummy felt empty from hunger. Noreen, one of my beloved 4C nurses, called it a "chemo cough." It would only cease once I ate.

This particular coughing fit was different from the ones I had before. My stomach felt sour, as though I was about to vomit. My eyes teared up as I took a step over to the edge of the curb. Though I would rather avoid it, I was prepared to throw up off the sidewalk. I stood still and carefully breathed in and out for half a minute. To my surprise, my stomach settled. Once I gingerly stepped over to the stoplight without feeling any sudden bodily urge to puke, I crossed the street when the light turned green. When I got to Paola's car two blocks away, I fetched my nausea medicine along with her bottle of water.

After our yummy lunch, Paola and I hit the road. I had offered to drive the first half of our trip home. An hour into our drive home, my head began to roll forward. My eyelids felt heavier and heavier while I tried to focus on the road ahead. Drumming my fingers against the steering wheel to the music did not help me become more alert. Once I realized that I would not be able to shake off my tiredness, I turned to Paola. She was resting her head against the window. She looked at peace. I put my hand on her thigh.

"Sweetheart," I said. "I'm sorry, but I should pull over and let you drive. I'm feeling really tired."

"It's okay."

I pulled over at the next exit, and we pulled a quick switcheroo. Once behind the wheel, Paola turned to me after she sensed that I was looking at her. A faint grin spread across my face before I leaned over to kiss her. She smiled, then drove us back on the highway. I leaned my head against the window and slept.

I am convinced that most couples have singular moments when everything in their relationship seems to be good. But moments like those can be like mirages, clouding over the doubts, the bad elements of a relationship. Months later, I would look back at that weekend with veneration and cling to it like a dream I believed was possible between Paola and me.

"We"

FOR OUR SECOND go-around, the wait to see Dr. Jaworski was not so agonizing. A little over an hour. Time in the waiting room went whizzing by thanks to Rick; he let me borrow his Game Boy for my war against Mr. Hodgkins. My thumbs were going ninja on Tetris's hardest setting while other patients were called by their physicians.

Our meeting was not very fruitful. These checkups were exactly that—a time to convene in order to discuss any difficulties arising from chemotherapy, from having a cancerous mass bent on gobbling my blood cells. The issues I brought up were the more-than-usual bouts of soul-depleting insomnia, the superficial thrombosis on my left arm (the veins on my forearm had darkened and were beginning to resemble those of a heroin junkie), the unusual darkening of the skin around my knuckles (they looked like they were smudged in dust), and the sudden fragility of my fingernails (on a few occasions, the nail on my index finger bent and cracked as I used it to pry off my pinky ring, since that finger—for whatever reason—had grown fatter like the others on my right hand). Funky shit was happening to my body, but it wasn't *bad*.

There was one notable thing that came out of our meeting: Jaworski told me that *we* would decide if chemotherapy would be continued past the fourth cycle. The results of my PET scan, scheduled for late September, would inform *our* determination. I smiled when he told me this. It gave me a sense of empowerment.

And better yet, the end to this perplexing turn in my life was nearing.

An Addendum to That Crazy Night with Tagi

NEAR THE END of August, Tagi and I met up for dinner. We dined at the tapas restaurant we loved. Shortly after we sat down, pints of beer in front of us, Tagi told me I had made out with her on that crazy night in June when I stalked back home, eager to beat the pulp out of anyone.

I shook my head. I was incredulous.

"Shit. Paola will break up with me if she finds out."

Tagi grimaced, then sipped her beer.

"I'm sorry," she said.

"You don't have to apologize for that. I was drunk—but I'm sure I only did what I wanted to then."

After I inquired, Tagi told me I began to make out with her at the Little Baobab dance club. After we lip-wrestled, I told her that she should have my kid—if she ever wanted one someday. This was nothing new. I had drunkenly told her that on previous occasions. My reasoning was simple: with our brains, the kid was bound to be super brilliant *and* beautiful if it came out looking like her. Tagi always found this flattering.

I decided to treat the incident as a mistake of sorts. My love, affection, and deep admiration for Tagi bubbled to the drunken-conscious surface in the form of a desirous kiss. That could explain why I left Tagi that night. Perhaps I realized what I was doing—kissing a woman other than Paola—and fled, upset at myself for allowing that to happen. For allowing another relationship to be tainted.

I chose not to tell Paola.

Gym Rat

PAOLA AND I walked among the other suits leaving their Financial District offices after a day of work. Side by side, we walked to her gym a few blocks away. I was going to be her guest. She was going to put in a "light cardio workout"—whatever that meant. It had been years since I had gone to a gym (which I like to pronounce to rhyme with "lime," just like Homer Simpson did in the episode when he became a gym rat). She thought I should consider joining. Their membership promotion ended that day.

At the front desk, Paola flashed her membership card and handed a guest coupon to the smiley attendant. Once their desk staff was aware of a guest in their vicinity, one of their service managers—a flaxen-haired guy—fixed his sights on me. He walked around the desk to introduce himself. His name tag read "David." He gave me an enthusiastic handshake and smiled as if he were meeting his girlfriend's father for the first time. "I'm just gonna give ya a quick tour of our gym and all its facilities, all right?" he asked.

I grinned and gave Paolita an "I'll see you later" nod, then followed David down a flight of stairs.

"Why are you considering a gym membership with us?" David asked when we got to the bottom of the stairs. We stood before a set of double doors that opened into a bright gym. A group of burly men stood behind him, clenching their jaws while they lifted barbells.

I told him that I felt I needed a good sweat every once in a while. I didn't tell him that I thought this would be a healthy practice since I was getting cytotoxic drugs injected into my body.

"This is our basement area where we keep our free weights and body-building machines," he said as we stepped into the room. He swiveled toward me with his hands on his hips. "Are you looking to bulk up? Add some definition to your muscles?"

"Oh, not right now."

"Okay. But why not?"

His line of unexpected questioning was flustering me. I was not sure why he was asking those questions. It almost seemed like he was challenging me—the presumably brainy, out-of-shape, white-collar tool—to embrace and unleash the inner hulk beneath my button-down veneer. But then I figured that he was just trying to appear attentive to unique, special me.

I decided to be honest with him. Keep it verdadero. My response would make this routine spiel a bit more memorable. So I told him I was undergoing chemo. Getting it shot into my arms. That it had kind of fucked them up, which is why I didn't think it was such a hot idea to do any heavy lifting while I underwent chemotherapy.

"Oh—" he said in response. His salesman grin was gone. "I'm sorry to hear that."

"Don't worry about it, man," I said with a nonchalant flick of my hand. "That's why I'm considering a membership—so I can sweat that shit out."

We walked up to the floor where they kept their cardiovascular workout machines. David shook my hand and told me to enjoy my workout.

Once I got out of my workday getup and into my jogging shorts and tank top, I walked around the rows of cardio machines until I saw Paola. She was by a corner of the gym, working out on an elliptical, a machine she had mentioned many times before. She was a curious sight. I had never seen her wearing sweat pants with her curly hair tied back in a ponytail. Her arms and plump legs were moving back and forth in a slow walking motion while she hovered over the ground in place. Paolita stared at a television tuned to CNN. Her iPod headphones were entrenched in her ears. On several occasions, she had told me she needed to work out more because she was "fat." I always scoffed at this word. Right then, I wished I could give her a big hug.

Instead, I snuck up behind her to pinch one of her butt cheeks. Paola whipped her head around. I giggled after realizing that I had startled her. (At her flat, I occasionally hid by the stairwell in the hallway to reach out and scare her when she walked out of the bathroom. I scared her good a few times; we got a kick out of it.) She shook her head and took out an earphone.

"You having fun?" I asked, looking up at her.

"Oh, tons, especially after my boyfriend sneaks up from behind to scare me!"

I laughed.

"I'll be over there, trying out those gizmos." I pointed toward the rows of gym denizens pedaling on exercise bikes and jogging on treadmills.

I hopped up on one of the exercise bikes. After I adjusted the seat height, I futzed around with its buttons while I listened to my "punk as fuck" iPod playlist. Once I got the hang of its settings, I took in my surroundings. The gym struck me as this incredibly strange place where a flock of half-naked people congregated to collectively sweat—even strain—through a series of motions that they silently repeated, again and again and again, on rows of identical machines. And it was out in the open for anyone to see. I felt like I was high as I looked around at this unfamiliar setting. This strange trip continued later when I stepped up on a treadmill. Over the years, I had become accustomed to an occasional trot around the neighborhood—up and down the steps and hills at Dolores Park or zigzagging and bounding around people on busy 24th Street as if I were Barry Sanders running a practice drill through the hood. It was disorienting to run in place on the treadmill, overlooking the street below. I was like the human equivalent of a mouse running in a wheel amid this urban landscape!

After my light workout, I walked over to David's work area. My tank top was drenched in sweat. I told him I wanted to sign up. I took a seat at his desk for our transaction dance. While he input my personal info into his computer, I leaned back in my chair with my hands clasped behind my head.

Throughout much of my adult life, I made fun of people who went to gyms. Like my professor, Wesley, I figured that most people who frequented gyms lacked imagination, a sufficiently interesting internal life. But there I was, sneaking in to be among them. I was proud that I was capable of swiftly adapting my ways in the face of this bewildering malady that was ushering change into my life.

Leaning back in my chair, I grinned while I watched David staple together my paper work.

Saint Mary's, Here I Come!

THE FIRST DAY of September was also the first day of fall semester classes. I put in a few hours of writing grants at the West Oakland office before I cycled over to the BART station to catch the afternoon train that would get me to school on time. Instead of disembarking at the Orinda station like I typically would, I rode the train to Lafayette. I wanted to cycle up the beauteous nature trail to school, the one I had daydreamt about throughout the summer.

I pedaled through Lafayette's posh downtown area over to the trail. One of my fight-cancer songs, Metallica's triumphant "Cyanide," blared from my headphones. It felt like a dream was coming true. I had wanted this moment to happen so badly. And it was! It really was! The ride along the Lamorinda hillside was just like I remembered it. Along the way, my bicycle odometer hit the six-thousand-mile mark. Most of those miles were notched in the city.

Once I turned into campus, sweat dripping off my chin, I was surprised I didn't feel a slew of intense emotions like I imagined I would. For the most part, I just felt really happy. I was too wrapped up in making it to class on time to come close to feeling emotional about the moment I had seized. I couldn't be late. My manuscript was being workshopped! It was something my classmates had never seen—the first chapters I drafted for this memoir.

After I locked my bike, I walked over to the back of Dante Hall, the stately white adobe building where our creative writing classes were held. Many of my classmates sat and gabbed on the stone benches beneath the wide, embracing branches of the tree that lorded over the lawn. My fellow second-year classmates greeted me as I stepped over to them, wiping sweat from my face with a hand towel. I was wearing shorts. My tank top was covered in sweat. Christine, one of my fellow nonfiction classmates, asked if I had cycled to school.

"Yup!" I said. I felt like a bad ass.

"Wow, that's great!" she said. "How are you feeling?"

"Pretty good. I can tell that I'm a little out of shape because it took me a little longer than usual to get here. But I feel great."

For workshop, I had submitted a twenty-page manuscript during our orientation the prior Sunday. To my delight, everyone really dug it, especially my fellow second-year classmates who were familiar with my work. Many of my fellow Nonfictionistas remarked at how "Juan" the writing was. The parenthetical asides. The manic, humorous tone. Wesley grinned and seconded them. In the hour we spent discussing my submission, my classmates almost unequivocally praised it. The one thing that was debated was my use of footnotes. More than half of the class was in complete support of how I was using them as a mixture of quips, tangents about my personal life, or as a place on the page where I could share medical information to accentuate the main text. A few classmates felt the footnotes should only provide medical facts. Other than that, my peeps had few things to criticize. I couldn't believe it. It was one of those rare workshops where little to nothing is criticized.

After class, one of the new students, Justine, came over to chat. She told me that she found it inspiring that I was bicycling to school and writing about my disease while I battled it. I blushed from her praise and thanked her. The handwritten comments on my stack of manuscripts were similarly supportive. (I have kept Wesley's note about my submission; it's tucked away in a drawer like an award I won.) It left me buzzing the rest of the evening. Probably the entire week.

With such encouragement, this memoir became my thesis. And I began to believe that I *could* create something beautiful from this mess.

Girlfriend Goes Wrong

A MINUTE AFTER Paola picked me up from my home, she asked if I could take the wheel. We were driving up the hill on Guerrero Street where the road looks like a speed ramp to the sky. We were on our way to Scott's abode in Oakland for our afternoon writing-group meeting. Our group was going to critique one of his submissions along with a twenty-page manuscript I had submitted.

"Why do you want me to drive?" I asked Paola as we approached the top of the hill. The surrounding Mission District and the city's downtown sprawled out before us.

"Because I haven't read your submission yet," she said with a demure voice.

I huffed. A few seconds later, I huffed again, shaking my head.

"Fuck that!" I said. "I'm not going to drive your car so you can read my submission. You should have already done that by now."

I stared at the cars in front of us. My eyes felt like lasers that could slice the windshield.

"Why didn't you read it during the week? Or yesterday? I uploaded it a week ago, Paola."

"I know, I know."

"What have you been doing all this time? I mean, I don't want to be some fucking asshole boyfriend. I don't expect you to be all interested in *every single thing* that I'm writing, and I don't expect you to treat me any differently than anyone in our group, but then, at the same time, I would *think* that if there was *any* person's submission you would care about, just a little bit more, it'd be mine. I don't think I'm asking for anything unreasonable here. I know that *I* treat everyone's submission equally. But if I tried to help a little more for anyone's, it'd be yours, because that's how I want to show you that I care about you."

A tense silence enveloped us while she drove to the freeway. Then, we received text messages from Scott. Our other group member, Lisa, could not attend. The meeting was canceled.

Paola turned the car around. Both of us were hungry. We rode down Valencia Street without saying a word. I was still fuming. Paola did her best to fill that silence by asking questions, such as what kind of food I would like to eat. I gave curt responses.

Before we started dating in early March, we hung out at cafés to read and write for our classes. Sometimes we went to her home if the café was too noisy. As the days became weeks, I found myself becoming fond of her. She was an educated, ambitious young Latina—an anomaly in San Francisco. For her undergraduate studies, she left her tiny Eastern Washington hometown to study at Vanderbilt. That was admirable and gutsy in my book. Shit, it took me nearly twenty-five years before I summoned the will to live on my own. After she graduated from Vanderbilt, Paola took internships at newspapers in Kansas City (she was proud to tell our writerly friends that the *Kansas City Star* was the paper Hemingway once wrote for), Baltimore, Detroit, Fort Worth, and Seattle before settling in Lafayette, California—the uppity town close to Saint Mary's. She completed her graduate studies while working full-time as a reporter *and* was part of a writing group that met weekly—a group she started. To boot, she *was* a talented writer; she wrote clear, succinct prose that I told her I would kill for.

But it had been four months since Paola graduated from Mills College. She was not writing. And we were no longer having our "writing dates" at cafés like we used to. Over those four months, it irked me, more and more. I was disappointed to find that she was not devoted to writing like I was, yet I was not sure *why* it should bother me in the first place. (Dealing with cancer was a *far* more urgent preoccupation.)

But once I became a part of her writing group, once I saw her attempt to speed-read my manuscript on a twenty-to-thirty-minute drive to Oakland, I could see that she was not quite the super ambitious, put-together person I thought she was. That's when Paola fell off this lofty pedestal on which I had held her up, when this dream I had of us began to crack.

The Disaster That Was Seattle

THERE ARE TWO things I remember about our flight to Seattle. The one moment I have replayed in my mind the most is the smile that Paola had when our plane rolled into the terminal. I did not ask why she was grinning. I figured she was happy to have me sitting beside her. For the first time, she was bringing a guy to spend time with her family. At that moment, I was not oblivious to the importance of that moment for Paola or myself.

The second moment I remember is the one "favor" Paola asked for our trip. She asked me not to tell her family I had cancer. Her siblings didn't know I had lymphoma. At least we didn't think so.

"Okay, but why?" I asked, furrowing my brow, recoiling inside. It was the first time I wondered if she felt embarrassed or disconcerted to be dating a guy who had such a bodily glitch.

"Because it'll probably be awkward, and I don't think they have to know."

It felt wrong to hide something I did not want to. Owning my disease was a major facet of my counteroffensive against Mr. Hodgkins. I didn't want to feel like a victim. I didn't want to feel like I had something bad to hide. Nevertheless, I could understand where Paola was coming from. This disease of mine put us both in awkward social situations, such as navigating a weekend visit with her family. And like me, she was apparently certain that this dark, cancer-shrouded period in my life would be exactly that—a period in my life. It would not be the End, like an unfinished sentence coming to a halt. I *would* survive. Her siblings didn't need to know because *there would be* a next time. And I wouldn't be holding Death's hand then.

The main reason Paola and I flew to Seattle was to attend her friend's Mexican wedding. It was my idea to accompany her. Paola had mentioned the wedding months before; it happened to fall on a non-chemo weekend. She was surprised that I wanted to go. She knew I wasn't fond of weddings in general.* Plus, I wanted to see more of Seattle. I believed it was a possibility that we would move there someday if our relationship lasted.

Paola's brother, Jesús, picked us up from the airport that Thursday evening. He had a sleek BMW for a ride. His buddies, Reñe and Alex (who I would later find out were his frat brothers at the University of Washington), sat in the backseat. After we had a jovial dinner at a Mexican restaurant in West Seattle, we drove to the town house Jesús and his sister, Rosa, owned.

Rosa and their spunky cousin, Cristina, greeted us at the door. We exchanged hugs and greetings. They introduced me to their adorable dogs—a teeny-tiny Chihuahua and a young, muscular pit bull mix named Rocco. (I liked to say his name in my Scooby Doo voice.) Paola, Jesús, and Jesús's bros wanted to hit the town. I was exhausted from a week of school and work—and I'd had my eighth infusion the Friday before—but I was determined to join them even though I practically had to peel myself off their couch.

Before long, the Boys, Paola, and I were back in the car. I had changed out of the dress clothes I had worn all day. Alex sat next to me in the backseat. As we rode out of West Seattle, I could see the city's skyscrapers off in the distance. That sight gave me my second wind. I

---

* Once I graduated from film school, I worked as a videographer and editor for two years. During that time, I must have filmed over fifty weddings and edited between fifty to sixty weddings. From those experiences, I came away with the impression that many of the weddings I witnessed were merely elaborate obligatory events whose main intent was to please the bride and groom's loved ones rather than to truly celebrate their love. And I often had the feeling that the brides cared more about having a lavish celebration that matched the fantasy they have been taught to dream of since they were girls instead of being genuinely in love with their partner. Too often, the wedding celebration felt like some big item to mark off their list of Things to Accomplish in Life.

Weddings seem gluttonous to me. A grand self-masturbatory event like few others. I know a former bridal store employee and musician who played at weddings, and they feel much the same way. I believe ritual *is* important, but it has always seemed nonsensical to me to spend a shitload of money—even go into debt—for a one-time event. I would much rather devote that money toward traveling to new places with my love, or toward something far more practical.

was excited to go out in the town that two of my favorite writers, Tom Robbins and Sherman Alexie, proudly call home.

But then Alex began to dominate the conversation in the car with his booming, nasally voice. He conversed with Jesús and Paola while Reñe and I sat quietly in the back. I stared out at the dark river water when we crossed the West Seattle Bridge, pretending to be fixated on it so I wouldn't have to engage with Alex. He laughed aloud at practically *anything* he said. I can't remember anything he said during that ride, but he would laugh aloud at something like, "Hey Jesús, remember those hot dogs we ate at the fair last year? Man, those things were *big*, JAJAJA!" It was beyond annoying to hear him laugh at something that was not inherently funny. To make matters worse, Paola cackled along with him from time to time. Reñe tittered to keep the bosom-buddyness rolling, but I wasn't having it. Within a matter of minutes, I felt like a prisoner in that backseat, as though I had been whisked off to a plane of earthly inferno in which a short, gauge-out-my-eardrums-annoying-chatterbox Latino laughed at any goddamn thing that came out of his incessant trap. I brooded with a silence that must have baffled him.

While I gawked at the skyscrapers we passed, Alex nudged me in the side.

"Ya all right, bro?" he asked.

"Yeah, man," I said, praying—*fucking praying*—that the ride would be over soon.

We drove out to the University District, the Boys' old stomping ground. We walked into Earl's on the Avenue, a college bar where young-and-dumb-and-full-of-cum undergrads got their drunken training wheels. Some teenage-looking kids drank at the bar, staring at the college basketball game on the TV. I felt like a chaperone at a high school dance.

We ordered drinks and made our way to the back of the bar. The booths and tables in the dimly lit hall were teeming with more youngsters who looked like they had just graduated from high school. Paola stood across from me, her back against the wall. I leaned against a booth where a husky, bald dude sat with the only other people who resembled fully grown adults. the Boys stood to a side, staring at the stage. It was karaoke night.

After a song finished playing, a young man walked onstage.

"All right, give it up for Darcy, coming to the stage," he said into the microphone, his words booming through the bar. The crowd politely applauded.

The husky guy stepped out of the booth. He slammed into my shoulder, which nearly made me spill beer from my glass. Then a parade of youngsters walked between Paola and me. I had to clutch my pint to my chest so they wouldn't knock into it. Once they passed, I looked over at Paola with a slight scowl. She had an apprehensive expression. She could probably tell I was not enjoying myself.

Since the bar was loud with chatter, I had to lean forward to speak into her ear.

"I *really* don't like this bar," I said.

Paola looked over at Jesús. He had a faint grin as he stood next to his chums, pint glass in hand.

"Do you wanna leave?" she asked.

"Yeah."

Paola looked over again at her brother, then back at me. She gave a half-grin before she leaned back against the wall since more patrons had to brush past us.

A young blonde strutted onto the stage, and "Closer" by Nine Inch Nails began to play. *Oh dear god*, I thought. To my horror, she commenced to sing with a sense of drunken abandon that seemed more of an advertisement to any horny straight guy in the bar. Her singing was ghastly. Someone might as well have dropped a turd in my drink. When the chorus played, she stepped out to the edge of the stage. She looked down at two guys sitting at a table. She sang the chorus as if she were the hottest woman alive, ready to bang them both in the nearest available stall.

I'd had enough.

I stalked past Paola without saying a word.

At the bar, I ordered a shot of Wild Turkey and knocked it back. It burned my throat, made the hairs on my arms stand up. I hung my head over the counter, then stared vacantly at the college hoops game for a minute or so. I didn't know what to do. The scene at the back of the bar was nauseating. I couldn't just stay at the bar while Paola, Jesús, and his friends wondered where I was. Wondered what the fuck was wrong with me.

If I had been home, I would have simply left.

But I was trapped.

I took a deep breath and walked back.

The young girl was "singing" the final part of the song. the Boys continued to look over the crowd with nostalgia-laden grins. It was apparent that they wanted to stay. I guess they still yearned to frequent bars where the *Girls Gone Wild* crew might show up.

Paola looked concerned when I walked up to her.

"Paola, I really don't want to be at this bar," I said. "This is—fucking abysmal. Standing here and listening to stupid shit like this is *not* my idea of fun."

"Well, what do you wanna do?"

"I just wanna get outta here!" I said, throwing up my hands. "I'm sorry, I don't wanna come across like some snotty guy, but I don't like being at a loud, annoying bar like this. This is what I did when I was an undergrad, man."

The song ended. The crowd applauded while Paola walked over to her brother. I felt bad, essentially demanding that we leave the bar. While they spoke, I looked away and sipped my drink. A minute later, Paola walked back.

"All right, let's go," she said.

Paola and I left the bar, then waited on the sidewalk until the Boys emerged.

"All right, so where do we go?" Jesús asked, looking at Paola.

"Well, Juan's feeling tired, and I think he wants to go home," she said, turning to me. I stood by her side, slightly apart from the group.

"No, no," I said, shaking my head, though I *would* have loved to have gone home. I felt a sudden surge of anger at Paola come over me. Why did she tell Jesús something I had not asked for? In the bar, I told her I was tired and should have stayed at their home, but I didn't tell her I wanted to head back. I didn't want to end their night out or have them drive me all the way back (though it had not occurred to me that I could have taken a cab back).

"I just couldn't stand that awful singing, that bar," I continued. "I was just hoping we could go somewhere that isn't so loud so we can hang out."

I had never been in such a situation before—being shown around town and asking to leave a place where I had been taken because I couldn't stomach it. Had I been in such a predicament before, I would

175

like to think that I'd have expressed gratitude to the person who took me there for leaving. But instead, I badmouthed a bar that they liked. My reaction at that moment is a bit puzzling to me now. Rather than act more humble and demure, I felt compelled—for whatever reason—to assert myself in front of Jesús. To show him I was confident and opinionated instead of just some polite boyfriend, as was expected of me for such a visit.

We walked into two nearby watering holes, but the Boys didn't seem to dig either one. We hopped back in the car. Alex continued his yammering until we arrived at a quaint brewery in an industrial part of Seattle.

Once we stepped through the swinging door, I took a deep breath of relief. Or perhaps rapture. It was a murky, spacious bar playing the loungy alternative rock I expected to hear in drizzly Seattle. Along the walls were cozy-looking couches. A group of people in their mid-twenties sat around one of the large mahogany tables in the middle of the room. A punk rocker with tall, spiked magenta hair conversed with the bartender. The bar had a decent selection of locally brewed beers including Mac & Jack's, Paola's favorite. We sauntered over to the bar. I continued to look around. There were two antique armchairs beside the entrance. A bearded fellow wearing a beret sat on one of them, reading a book beneath the warm pool of light from an antique lamp. And just like that, all the bullshit from earlier that day—feeling super stressed on the train ride from Moraga to the Oakland Airport because I was afraid I would miss our flight, the college bar, and the Agony That Was Alex—felt worthwhile. This is what I had hoped to find in Seattle—a place that fit into the dreary yet chillaxingly vibrant grunge universe I had fantasized about since high school, when I became obsessed with Nirvana. Looking around the bar, I thought, yup, I can be happy here.

Then Alex and Jesús ordered not one but two pitchers of beer.

Oh shit, I thought. It's gonna be one of *those* nights.

It must have been past midnight when we left the bar. I trailed behind the pairs: Paola and Jesús, Alex and Reñe. We'd chummed it up over a few games of pool and refills of my pint that I couldn't keep count of. Once we set foot on the sidewalk, my stomach took a turn for the queasy. It was sudden, unexpected. I lurched between two cars parked in front of the bar and vomited. Some of it splattered on the sides of my Chuck Taylor shoes. I had hoped that my public retching had gone unnoticed, but Alex and Reñe watched me emerge from the parked cars.

"Oh, dude, you drank too much!" Alex said. He slapped my back and guffawed.

My face felt hot like a cauldron ready to blow its lid. I was embarrassed, upset that my chemo-self seemingly couldn't handle this amount of liquor like it typically could. I was fucking pissed I couldn't explain myself by saying, "I have cancer, and I'm doing chemo—and I guess my body can't handle alcohol like it usually does." But Paola had asked me to keep that to myself, so I stared at the pavement all wobbly and kept my mouth shut.

On the car ride home, I sat captive in the same backseat spot next to Alex, behind Paola. They yakked and laughed it up while I kept to myself. I felt like a body of smoldering charcoal as we rode through the night.

At one point, Alex leaned between the two front seats. He was poking fun at Paola in a typically Mexican way. Their banter was like a murmur of laughter meshed with the car's droning motor. I wasn't paying much attention to what they were saying, but I seized the opportunity to smack the back of her seat in a passive-aggressive way, saying "Yeah, what were you thinking!" I hit it hard enough that Alex recoiled, said *whoa!*, and Jesús whipped his head back to glare at me. I knew I had done something wrong, so I looked away. A tense silence filled the car before Alex continued to yammer.

We stopped at a gas station to pick up a twelve-pack of Coronas. Reñe and Alex left to go to the pull-up window. I bent over in my seat, a piece of napkin in hand. I tried to wipe the vomit from my shoes with the faint light from the half-moon. It was no use. I couldn't rub it off the black canvas. Then I saw an air-water machine a few feet from the car.

I stepped out. I had no quarters in my wallet, but perhaps they didn't charge fifty cents to operate them in Washington? I grabbed the water hose and pressed the lever. A few drops dribbled out. I stalked back to the car, avoiding eye contact with Paola and Jesús.

"Were you trying to get it to work?" Paola asked as I took my seat in the back.

I was still angry at her, though I didn't entirely know why. And her question seemed utterly stupid, especially for someone whose profession required her to be observant.

(If that night had been edited like an episode of *Blind Date*, the editor would have created a countdown caption at the bottom of the television screen that read: "Juan and Paola's visit to Seattle to spend time with her family takes a disastrous turn in 3 . . . 2 . . . 1 . . .")

"What does it look like I was tryin' to fuckin' do?" I asked.

Neither of them said a word. (Our *Blind Date*–style episode would have been titled "How to Ruin Relations with Your Girlfriend's Siblings in One Weekend.") Instead, we stared out into the dark, barren field in front of us.

The next morning, I awoke to find myself curled on one of the couches in Rosa and Jesus's living room. Slits of piercing sunlight sliced through the blinds and curtains that covered the windows. Paola was asleep on the other couch. My eyes stung from lack of sleep. My forehead felt a tad singed. Quietly, I pushed the blanket off to go to the bathroom. Paola opened her eyes and watched me walk past her. I greeted her by shooting her a look. I was still pissed off—at her, I supposed—though I still could not articulate why.

In the dimly lit bathroom, I pissed with a sense of complete dejection. Thinking about all the booze I should not have drunk. The bad things I had done and said to Paola the night before. Once I realized how awful the night had turned out, I snickered at myself. I could have pissed on my feet, all over myself for all I cared. I had essentially done that the night before.

While I splashed water on my dehydrated face, I tried to figure out why I felt mad at Paola. I stood in front of the mirror and listened to the water run from the faucet. I realized I was mad at her because I had to keep my mouth shut while Alex laughed at me. I had to give that annoying fucker a pass because I couldn't tell him I had cancer, couldn't tell him that my digestive system did not seem to handle alcohol like it normally could after eight chemo-fucking-therapy infusions. Had I been able to explain that and put him in his place, would I have snapped at her?

But despite that, I was unable to keep that anger to myself, drunk and emotional like I was.

I had to take out my rage on something.

And too often, it was Paola.

Before I stepped out of the bathroom, I also realized that I was upset because I felt trapped the night before, stuck in a car beside Alex. I was upset at myself for going out to drink when I should have stayed home to rest. But those were my choices, each one of them: my choice to accompany Paola to Seattle; my choice to go out; my choice to drink throughout the night. Paola was not to blame for any of those actions. I was.

The anger I had carried over from the night before began to dissipate. I walked back to the living room. I said a distant good morning to Paola, then asked how she felt.

Later that Friday night, Paola and I drove out to Alki Point. Side by side, bundled up in our pea coats, we walked along the promenade. Across the bay, the lights from the Seattle skyline twinkled on the waters of Puget Sound. Earlier that day, Jesús, Paola, and I went out on the town. Per my request, we visited the Seattle Public Library where I giddily snapped picture after picture of their various floors. Then we strolled around Pike Place Market before we hit up Ivar's Acres of Clams, where I drained three happy hour beers on an empty stomach and made raunchy jokes and smacked the table a few times to be overly dramatic about something trivial in front of Jesús and a contingent of his friends who joined us. Sober or tipsy, these were things I did with a few of my friends if I was feeling playful and irreverent; they'd come to expect it, but I don't think I endeared myself to Paola's brother—dressed in dark jeans and a white Washington Huskies football jersey—with my antics.

The gentle sound of the lapping waves enveloped Paola and me as we walked out to a small pier. We finally had some time to ourselves.

"Paola, I'm really sorry about last night," I said. "I obviously had too much to drink, but that's no excuse for smacking the back of your seat like I did. That was completely passive-aggressive of me. I was angry at you."

"But why?" she asked. We sat on a cold bench that looked out over Puget Sound. I told her I was mostly angry at myself for drinking too much, and because I wasn't supposed to tell Alex I had cancer after he laughed at me. She understood.

Hands tucked into our coat pockets, we stared out to the skyline as a breeze blew.

"It's getting a little chilly, huh? You wanna get going?" Paola asked.

"Yeah, sure."

As we stood, an old woman walked by with her small dog.

"What I'm really sorry about are those awful words I said to you in the car, when we stopped at the gas station," I said. "I am really, really sorry for saying that, Paola. There's absolutely no reason that I should ever say such hurtful things to you."

"It's okay," Paola said in a tone that was far more forgiving than I expected or felt I deserved. She even reached out to hold my hand. Perhaps she knew how awful I felt about it. Or perhaps she was just tired of accepting my apologies. Hand in hand, we walked into a pool of streetlight on our way to the car.

"Are you going to apologize to my brother?"

"Apologize for what?"

"For what you did last night."

"That'd be awkward. I think me and your brother get along all right, but I don't really know him. We've never come close to talking about anything serious, so it'd be weird if I apologized to him for my actions. And really, if there's one person I should apologize to, to ask for forgiveness, it's you. Not him. And I've already done that."

My rationale seemed sound at the time, but I failed to understand how I *had* disrespected Jesús that night. By disrespecting Paola in front of him, I had done the same to him. I failed to see such an obvious truth then. And Paola did not pursue that matter further.

But my response to her question was not the most foolish thing I said that seemingly tranquil evening. Before we stepped into her sister's car, Paola and I took in the gorgeous view of Seattle one last time. With a chipper voice, I said, "I sure wouldn't mind moving here someday." She made an uncomfortable smile and gave a soft "hmmm." I didn't think anything of her curious reaction.

I also failed to see how badly I had already fucked up our relationship, especially by not apologizing to her brother. In short time, Jesús told Rosa about the horrible behavior he witnessed. Then their mother found out. And just like that, Paola's family despised me as if I were a low-life bum. Or a batterer.

And I had *no* clue.

Over

WITH A MOROSE expression fit for a wake, Paola stood at my front door on the night we returned from Seattle. My facial expression must have been equally grim. A few hours after we flew into Oakland on an early Monday morning flight, she left a voicemail that caused a heavy, sickening weight to sit in my stomach for the rest of the day. In her voicemail, once she got past formalities, Paola said, "I was wondering if you're free tonight because we need to talk."

Those words caught me off guard because everything seemed to be fine between us earlier that morning. At Tacoma-Seattle Airport, Jesús, Rosa, and Cristina woke up at 5:30 a.m. to drop us off. It was all smiles and hugs when we said good-bye at the unloading area. I exchanged hugs with Rosa, even Jesús, although our handshake-morphed-into-a-bro-hug was awkward. Jesús was reluctant to put his arm around me, but in my continued obliviousness to the mess I had made, I was not alarmed by his reaction. I thought I had righted the perilous beginning of our trip with a righteous time at her friend's wedding on Saturday, then a mostly chill Sunday that included a sunshiny walk to a nearby park with Paola, Rosa, and her pit bull. I was certain that the visit went over okay when Cristina gave me a warm hug and said, "Take care of yourself. Wow, I guess we'll see you again!" I smiled and replied, "Yeah, I'm sure I will," assured that another trip to visit them with Paola was a mere formality. Through it all, Paola grinned. She did not make any unusual ambivalent or anguished expression as though she was witnessing a scene that would never happen again between her family and me. During our flight and train ride into San Francisco, Paola never acted in a peculiar way to raise my concern.

Once I closed the front door behind me, Paola and I walked across Dolores Street to her car. We didn't say a word to each other. I became acutely aware of the sound of our footsteps on the quiet street. Before she opened the car door, she asked if we should go somewhere. With a resigned voice, I said it didn't matter where our conversation took place, that we might as well stay in her car where we would at least have privacy.

Once we settled into our familiar seats, I turned to Paola. She eventually turned to me.

"You know that my family is very important to me," she said.

"Yeah, I know that." I turned to stare at the car parked in front of us.

"I have to break up with you, Juan, because my family doesn't think I should be with you after our trip to Seattle."

I sighed. She began to cry.

Our breakup went on for about a half hour. She expressed her shock at the way I acted that Thursday night in Seattle in front of her brother. Like evidence to substantiate her decision, which I could not protest, she brought up the other ugly drunken episodes in our short time together: my thirtieth birthday, the night I called to tell her I wanted to kill someone, and her twenty-eighth birthday. All the while, I sat there with my hands cupped in my lap, staring at the glove box like a boy being lectured by an adult on all the bad things he had done. While Paola continued to cry, even blowing her sniffly nose, I felt withdrawn, like when my mother cried at our meeting with my oncologist. When I spoke, I did so with a low, measured voice.

The only time I felt myself rise out of that numb shell was when she told me that Jesús was afraid for her safety. He thought I was a violent person. That got a snicker out of me.

"Why does he think that?" I asked.

"Because you smacked my seat when we were in his car, and because you were slamming your hand on the table at the restaurant, Juan."

I shook my head in disbelief.

"I have never hit a woman, Paola," I said. This was partly true. I used to get in hitting fights with Carmen until we were in junior high. "I used to work at a domestic violence agency, for Christ's sake. How can he say I'm a violent person when he doesn't even know anything about me?"

By the end, Paola had blown her nose on a few tissues. It was heart-breaking to sit there and watch her wipe away her tears over someone like me. I didn't feel worthy of those tears. Soon after, we had little to say. It was time to leave.

"I just want you to know that I really regret that it's turned out this way," I said, looking down at my hands. "This is definitely not what I wanted for us. I want you to know I feel really sad right now, even though it may not show. I wish I could cry right now, but ever since I've been diagnosed, I've had a hard time expressing my sorrow. I just feel numb right now because I don't want to feel sad."

"I'm sorry it's turned out this way, too," Paola said with a sob that she stifled.

I leaned over the parking brake that we used to hold hands over. I put my arm around her back and let her tuck her face into my shoulder. We hugged tightly. Staring out the window to my house, I rested my chin on her shoulder, thinking to myself that I should be feeling more emotional.

"I'm sorry, Paola. I'm sorry," I whispered into her ear. She lifted her face. We pressed our cheeks together. I could feel her warm tears against my face. I kissed her teary cheek, wiped it dry with my hand, and left.

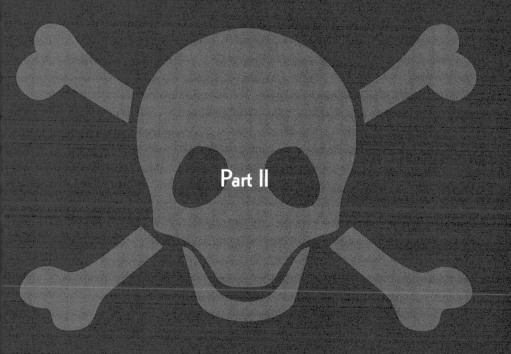

Part II

Bleeding Me

PAOLA'S ABSENCE LEFT a void in my everyday life. It shrouded the imaginary future I had begun to presume she would be a part of. I couldn't help but look back, again and again, at the terrible acts I had done during our relationship.

And I realized I had some problems.

Problems controlling my anger.

Problems handling alcohol.

(It's startling how long it took me to realize these issues, but I've often been a late bloomer about a number of things.)

Like the lone patron in a screening room inside my head, I replayed that living nightmare, that Thursday night in Seattle when I snapped at Paolita in front of her brother. I also screened the Friday morning when I arose from the couch and glared at Paola. It was punishing to relive those moments; it exacerbated the profound regret and shame I already felt. As I replayed each one, again and again, I thought to myself, *How could you say such things to someone you're supposed to love?* Or, *There you go again, fucking up another relationship. You sack of shit.* But the screenings were necessary. I was searching for an answer.

And I was struck with a thought: *It doesn't have to be this way.*

Since my childhood, my family left me alone whenever I was angry. If I wasn't in the haven of my room, I would stalk around our house. I would sulk and ignore the person I happened to be angry at (which was usually Carmen). It was not uncommon for me to fire some serious stink eyes at a particular loved one until I decided to not be so pissy. That's how I dealt with my anger.

I felt entitled to act that way—and it carried into adulthood, into my romantic relationships. For years, if my moodiness or anger ever became an issue, I would counsel my girlfriends by telling them that the best way to deal with me in such instances was to leave me alone. Leave me be, I would suggest, until those emotions would drain out of me. Then I could reason like a more rational person again.

When I played back that morning scene in the living room, I realized that there *must* be another way I could have handled that situation. All my life, I had come to believe this is *how I am when I'm angry*—a given I was born with like my black hair.

But I realized that it was *my choice* to react in that way.

I owed it to myself and to those I loved to learn a different, healthier way.

The day after Paola broke up with me, I did not want to talk to anyone. I wanted to drown myself in bleak music while I rescreened those regretful memories. But I *did* have to deal with other people, because I didn't want to skip work or school.

At my tiny office, I played the Metallica station on Pandora Radio. A song from their *Load* album came on. I had not heard it in years. The song was "Bleeding Me"—and it could not have been timelier. Alone at my desk, I felt the wearied, delicate opening chords to my core. The song's tone, its lyrics mirrored how I felt inside.

I had always dug the song. Hammett plays an astounding solo, and it is arguably the most anguished song that James Hetfield ever wrote. Undoubtedly one of his most personal. I had never understood the ordeal expressed through that song like I did then.[*] Staring at a corner of the computer screen, I sat there transfixed, listening to my life through one of their songs yet again.

That night, I came home and shut my bedroom door. With my headphones on, I sat at my desk and listened to the song with my eyes half-closed, whispering the lyrics to myself, imagining myself on a stage,

---

[*] A year later, I found an interview with James Hetfield in which he discussed "Bleeding Me." He said it was about his lifelong troubles with alcohol. It was validating and a relief to hear that. Throughout my life, I've had a propensity for getting a key song lyric completely wrong, then concocting an erroneous idea of what it's about. I was glad "Bleeding Me" wasn't about a gambling addiction or a sympathetic ode to hemophiliacs.

guitar in hand, singing it to a crowd (which might as well have been only myself—that edition of myself I did not want to be).

When Hetfield wailed the last verse before the band launched into the cathartic chorus, I began to choke up as though I was the one who had written the song.

Because that's what I wanted it to be.

My anthem.

Hallelujah

THE LATE-MORNING SUN shined through my office window, illuminating the yellow-beige walls of the massive Victorian that used to be a convent. I sat at my wooden desk, hunched over the keyboard, staring at the flat-screen monitor as I revised a grant proposal. Pandora was playing classic Motown songs from the Supremes station. The computer speakers crackled as they often did when my cell phone was about to receive a text or call. My phone vibrated in my pocket. It was a 415 number—a familiar-looking one. I pushed my seat out and reached over to close the door. Before I took the call, I lowered the volume on the speakers. I took a breath. I had been expecting this call all week. It was Wednesday, two days before my tentatively scheduled ninth infusion. It was the verdict—whether I would continue chemotherapy or not.

"This is Juan," I said into the phone.

It was Bryn, the oncology nurse.

"I'm calling because Dr. Jaworski is running around, busy with appointments today," she said. "But he wanted me to tell you that after reviewing your recent PET-scan results, which came back great, and comparing them with the one taken back in June, he's determined that the treatment has been effective and you don't have to come in this Friday."

"So I'm done with chemo?" I asked, a ridiculously huge grin coming over me. I swiveled my chair to face the window. It looked out over the mighty oak tree that loomed over the Center's backyard.

"Yup, you're done!"

I tittered.

191

"That's great news. Thank you, Bryn."

"Dr. Jaworski will meet and discuss with you the hand-off in treatment with Dr. Kirsch when you have your oncology appointment next Wednesday, okay?"

"Okay!"

"Thanks, Juan. We'll see you then."

I lifted my head and stared out to the tree's rich foliage, to the bright-blue sky beyond. I bowed my head as my eyes filled with tears, the sun's warmth shining all over me.

MONDAY NIGHT FOOTBALL, October 5, 2009. Green Bay Packer legend Brett Favre was facing his old team for the first time since he joined their rival, the Minnesota Vikings. It was gonna be a helluva game. Both teams were potential title contenders and bitter division rivals. The game promised to provide its share of emotions and drama given Favre's storied history with his former team. Although I was a huge football fan, I rarely ever marked my calendar for a game. (I have always been drawn to the combination of brute force and calculating strategy the game entails.) But this was one game I noted.

I was in Fremont that weekend. Before I received word from the oncology nurse, it was supposed to have been one of my chemo weekends, but I visited since my parents had grown accustomed to having me over every two weeks. And I liked being there, too, especially when Negrita curled up on my lap while I read in the living room. Life was more relaxing with them instead of in the bustling Mission.

My parents had invited Tío José Luis and Heide over for dinner. Mom was excited to tell them I was done with chemotherapy. They gave me congratulatory hugs when they left. I was glad to soak up the happiness and collective relief we felt.

The Monday Night game seemed like one worthy of watching with a crowd at a bar. I invited my dad to join me—at least for the first half—at this dive called Roamers. The bar was down the main road from my parents' home. We drove over before the game started.

Dad and I hunkered down on stools near one end of the bar. The Temptations' "My Girl" played from the jukebox. Mi papito was bundled up in his old-man khakis and a blue-and-gray rain jacket that covered his button-down shirt. Sitting on the stool beside him, I felt like a kid teetering in oversized boots to go fishing with his dad (although we never came close to doing anything like that; my parents are not outdoorsy types). Though my dad had seen me drunk a number of times—and certainly heard stories of the locuras I was capable of—it was the first time we had ever gone to a bar together. As expected, there were few people at the neighborhood bar: a stocky Latina with a booming, ragged voice; two dudes in their mid-twenties with Oakland A's hats flanking her sides; and two middle-aged men—one with a big beer gut who looked like he had just finished a day working at a warehouse and another guy who picked at a bowl of stale yellow popcorn (the staple snack at any respectable blue-collar dive bar in Fremont).

The bartender took our order—a bottle of Negra Modelo for my pop and a pint of Sierra Nevada for me. When the bartender hit us up for payment, I put my hand out and said, "Don't worry, Dad. I got it." We clanged our glasses and said "cheers."

Dad and I watched as Favre's Vikings jumped out to a lead in front of their roaring Metrodome fans. He sipped his beer while a few more patrons stepped into the bar. A rail-thin, middle-aged man with wire-rimmed glasses that gave him the faint look of a child porn enthusiast sat alone at a small table beside the bar. He muttered and cursed whenever the Vikings' defense sacked Favre's successor, Aaron Rodgers.

As the game continued into the second quarter, the other patrons got rowdier. Their shouts and guffaws filled the lounge. When I polished off my pint, I noticed that my dad was not even half done with his beer. Amid the shouting from the other patrons (*GET HIS ASS!*), my pop sat quietly, his eyes fixed disinterestedly on the television on our side of the bar. He had a curious expression on his face that I had not expected.

"You okay, Dad?" I asked.

"Yeah, yeah," he said.

"You wanna get going soon?"

"Nah, no son. Go ahead, get yourself another beer."

"Are you sure? We can leave whenever you want."

"Nah, go ahead."

I ordered another pint, then left for the restroom. On my way back to my stool, I was struck by how timid, how out of place my pop appeared. He was hunched over the counter, his arms tucked together.

I figured he would have enjoyed leaving the house to do something with just me. But I seemed to have figured wrong. He almost seemed scared to interact with any of the folks at the bar—as though they were unpredictable creatures to be careful of.

My dad gave a faint grin when I sat next to him, patting him on his back.

Given all the shameful memories I had been fixating on in regard to alcohol and how it brought out the worst in me, I began to look at the other bar patrons as though they were almost a different species altogether. Their sudden dramatic shouts and subsequent predictable cursing in reaction to a play—such as an incomplete pass on third down—seemed bizarre. Almost frightening. It gave me pause. And just like that, those bottles of alcohol behind the counter, placed out of our reach, even the glass of beer in front of me, looked like dangerous substances to be weary of. They were capable of inducing these beasts within us.

My dad and I left soon afterward.

El Loco versus Mr. Hodgkins

INT. LOCKER ROOM—NIGHT

Mr. Hodgkins, dressed in his tuxedo, stands next to a balding, musta-chioed man, Mean Gene Okerlund. They both face a large Panavision television camera. Donning a black suit, holding a microphone, Oker-lund stares at the woman wearing a headset. She stands beside the cameraman. Okerlund nods when she points at him. She holds her fingers up in a silent countdown—three, two, one—before the red lamp on top of the camera turns on.

MEAN GENE OKERLUND

We are just minutes away from our career-ending match between "El Loco," Juan Alvarado Valdivia, and the gentleman standing beside me, Death himself, Mr. Hodgkins.

Okerlund stretches his hand out to Mr. Hodgkins.

MEAN GENE OKERLUND

Mr. Hodgkins, I've got to ask you, just what exactly is it that you have against El Loco? You've come into his life and, without exagger-ation, turned his world upside-down, casting a dark pall over it. Tell me, why him?

Mean Gene holds the microphone up to Mr. Hodgkins. Hodgkins stares back at the camera with an indifferent expression that Camus would have envied.

MR. HODGKINS

It's like this, Okerlund. I have nothing personal against the man. We simply crossed paths—and it is my job to ensure that he suffers the consequences. It is nothing more than that. He's the one who has taken it personally—the flawed, vengeful human that he is. I do not hold that against him. Nevertheless, my objective is to annihilate him. And I will.

Mr. Hodgkins stalks out of camera view. Okerlund watches him leave, then turns back to the camera after a long, dramatic pause.

MEAN GENE OKERLUND

And now let's go to Sean Mooney, who's standing by with El Loco, Juan Alvarado Valdivia.

INT. INTERVIEW ROOM—NIGHT

SEAN MOONEY

All right, thanks Gene. El Loco is in rare form tonight. He's been pacing this room ever since I got here.

While Mooney stands in front of the camera, Juan—in El Loco gear— paces behind him in front of a black curtain. He pumps his arms and gives an occasional menacing snarl to the camera. Earthy-brown and green-colored tassels are tied around his wrists and bronzed biceps. A mask bearing the same colors has been painted on his face. His arms, chest, and modest paunch are varnished in body oil. They glare beneath the studio lights. Besides the tassels, the only things he wears are tasseled brown boots and short green trunks.

SEAN MOONEY

El Loco—I don't think I've ever seen you this amped up before a fight! And you're always roaring, running full speed into the ring and yanking on those ropes as though a lightning bolt was coursing through your veins.

El Loco grabs Mooney by the collar.

EL LOCO

Well, what can ya expect, Mooney? This is the fight of my life!

He shoves Mooney back, snarling at the camera.

EL LOCO
Of course I'm pumped up! This is it—this is *fucking it* for me or that punk, Mr. Hodgkins. Well, no one gets to take my life except me!

Juan's mouth drops. His brows furrow. He looks away, ashamed to have stumbled upon this truth before a live television broadcast.

He turns back to the camera, shaking his head violently as if he were trying to wake from a daze. Mooney leans his head back frightfully. He holds the microphone out to El Loco as he points at the camera.

EL LOCO
You fucked with the wrong man, Hodgkins. You fucked with the wrong man.

Juan turns his back to the camera. He cranes his head back and lifts his clenched fists up high. He roars, then pounds his chest like a gorilla.

EL LOCO
Just take a look at my trunks. It says it all, right there, baby.

Juan cackles. He pumps his arms. The camera zooms down to the green trunks covering his butt. Mr. Hodgkins's head, with his signature derby hat atop, is stitched on them. Below it reads: YOUR ASS IS MINE!

El Loco roars and dashes out of the room.

Break Up to Make Up

OVER A WEEK had passed since Paola broke up with me. We decided to meet up on a Wednesday evening to discuss our relationship. We met at Socha Café. It was a fitting choice. Though we never really had a song as a couple, Socha was without question our place. It was the café where our friendship and love for each other had sprouted.

Paola and I met in the back room, which was covered with photos and sprawling digital mixed-media prints from local artists. She sat on a padded bench, bundled up in jeans and a jacket. She wore dark red lipstick, which struck me as unusual. After I placed my cup of hot chocolate on our small table, we hugged and sat across from each other.

Once we got past formalities, I started by telling her I had come to realize I had some personal issues I needed to take care of if I wanted to have a healthier relationship with her, or anybody. I told her I thought I had a problem controlling my anger. Having lymphoma had exacerbated that personal issue because I had never felt so angry in my entire life. What made it worse was that there was no one to rightly direct it at. I told Paola I had searched online for anger management books. I had already ordered one. Since Paola had criticized me before for reacting negatively to many situations, I did my best to sound optimistic when I told her I was determined to read them in short time. And I was. Other than regaining my good health, my attempt to improve my behavior was the most critical goal in my life. I believed I could salvage our relationship. I believed I could become a better partner.

Once those points about my anger were covered, I steered our conversation to my drinking.

"I've come to a point in my life where I'm not sure if I want to drink anymore," I said. "It's the first time I've even considered quitting. After our trip to Seattle, I think I've reached a point where I'm not sure if alcohol has brought more harm and suffering into my life than good."

This was the first time I was expressing these brand-new thoughts. My voice was inflected from the weariness I felt. Paola looked at me with a sympathetic expression, as if she was ready to reach over to hold my hand.

"I think quitting altogether would be the easier thing to do," I said. "I think the bigger challenge would be figuring out how to control my drinking, which I think I'm capable of. If we decided to get back together, I could use your help. If we were out, say, drinking with friends and you saw me getting out of hand, you could tell me—with a caring tone—that I was drinking too much and should stop."

Paola frowned.

"No, I can't support that," she said. "I don't think that should be my responsibility."

I was thrown back by her unwillingness to help. When I drank during her birthday and in Seattle, it's not like I went out those nights with the intention of getting hammered. It's hard to explain without it sounding like I am completely making excuses, but when I reach a certain level of drunkenness it's like a switch flips inside and I can't stop myself from drinking. All along, that was a sign of being an alcoholic, but for years I thought I could overcome it. Control it. Or at least keep it to minimum, which is why I asked for Paola's help. But I could understand why she was unwilling to be the drink police. A few months later, I would understand that her stance was absolutely correct.

Paola then told me that she had made calls to close friends and family. She discussed our hardships with them. From those conversations, she came to realize that relationships are tough work. In the past, whenever her fleeting relationships had taken any difficult turn, she typically fled. During our brief time together, she had come to understand that good relationships are not like the fairy-tale romances from the romantic comedies she loved. Work was needed every day to keep them healthy.

I nodded because I was coming to understand this as well. And I was hopeful Paola would give us a second chance.

Throughout our respective lives, Paola and I hadn't been the long-term relationship type. Not like my sisters who were rarely ever single throughout their adulthoods. Back then, my longest relationship was one and a half years—which included four breakups before we parted ways for the final time. Otherwise, the longest continuous relationship I had lasted only eleven months. Before we dated, Paola's longest relationship in her twenty-eight-year life was five months. She told me she had intimacy issues because of her father's sudden death when she was a teenager; she was afraid of getting close to someone because she was afraid of being abandoned (which made it all the more baffling why she kept dating a guy with lymphoma). Without a doubt—if I could have been an objective party—we would have been the last couple to bet on lasting for a long time. Like a duo of talented sprinter horses gunning to win a long race.

I assured Paola that whether or not we decided to try and make things work out, I was going to work on my personal issues. "But I think you need to step up and do your part to make our relationship better, too," I said.

When I said this, Paola recoiled slightly in her seat. Her eyes narrowed. She looked like she was about to cross her arms.

"I've realized why it has bugged me so much that you haven't been writing since you graduated," I said. "That's why *I fell for you*, Paola. That's what made you different from all the other girlfriends I've ever had. You were artistic, even a writer like me."

She hadn't heard this before—that this was the dream I had for us.

"The moment I really became smitten with you was when I saw you read at Mills, when you wore your red dress."

Paola nodded. She looked a bit morose. I brought up the writing group meeting when she didn't read my submission. I told her I had a right to be angry at her because she disrespected me by not reading my manuscript, by disregarding my writing. She knew it was one of the most meaningful aspects of my life.

Paola told me she understood.

"Well, I want to feel more special when we spend time together," Paola said. "I would like us to do more than just hang out at my place. I want to dress up and go on more dinner dates. To the movies—and I want to go out dancing more often."

I told her I would like that, too (though I was not thrilled with the idea of going out to dance more often).

We left the café when it closed at 10 p.m. An air of uncertainty hung between us. We still needed to reach some commitment, some conclusion, so we walked down the street to El Rio. At the bar, we sat by ourselves at a corner on the back patio. When I asked where she stood, Paola said she could only commit to dating. One thing at a time to see how things would transpire. To see if our relationship could improve. I was pleased. I even joked that we were essentially "on probation," though Paola didn't find that comment as amusing as I had hoped.

And so, we were sorta kinda back together again.

Halt the Celebration
(and Please Return Your Party Hats)

A FEW DAYS later, I awoke to find a voicemail message from the receptionist at UCSF's Radiation Department. She informed me that my appointment the following week with Dr. Kirsch had been canceled. It was a doozy of an awakening—an utterly befuddling one. A trucker-strength cup of coffee could not have awoken me more as I leapt out of bed muttering, *What. The. Fuck.* Never in my life as a resident of this modern world where hunting and gathering food entails finding my wallet and walking down the street had I felt such an instinctual desperation for my life. It had been exactly three weeks since my cancer-infected body had received a chemotherapy infusion. In theory, the cancerous mass—if it was still active, like a brush fire in my chest—was now growing instead of shrinking; that was the notion behind continuous treatment—we could not allow the disease to continue to spread throughout my body. So when I heard that my appointment with Dr. Kirsch was canceled, the man who would oversee the final leg of treatment that would hopefully save my hide, I might as well have been a wind-up doll that had its operating knob wound to ¡¡¡DESESPERADO!!!, sending my arms flailing, eyes bulging, pupils bouncing everywhere like Super Balls while I yelled and ricocheted from wall to wall.

But instead of screaming my head off in panic, I called the receptionist back. She told me I had to meet with the oncology department at San Francisco General before any transition to radiation treatment could take place. Now, this was particularly confusing because *I had met* with my oncologist, Dr. Jaworski, *two days before*. He told me I was done with chemotherapy! And I received no further communication from their department since that meeting.

I called the oncology department. I left a message with the oncology nurse, then adopted a cordial business veneer in writing an e-mail to Dr. Jaworski, which must have sufficiently glossed over the desperation bubbling inside me. (For example, when I wrote, "I can't miss that appointment with Dr. Kirsch," the font type—if it were to reflect my emotions—should have been in bold with an eighty-point font.)

Dr. Jaworski called me later that morning. He explained *his* sudden decision to cancel radiation treatment and cease chemotherapy after four cycles of treatment. (All his prior talk about making such a decision together turned out to be as hollow as a politician's campaign promise.) He told me the PET scan taken back in June clearly demonstrated that my cancerous mass was not large enough to merit this additional treatment. Thusly, he was reluctant to expose me to further unnecessary treatment that would only increase my chances of developing cancer again, or something nastier—like leukemia or myeloma.

Once I met that wall, I e-mailed the man who both of my oncologists spoke of with reverence:

From: Juan Alvarado Valdivia
To: Richard Kirsch
Subject: Regarding the cancellation of my radiation treatment
          with you
Date: Fri, Oct 9, 2009, 12:04 p.m.

Hi Dr. Kirsch,

I met with you back on 6/16/09; I was then a patient of Dr. Attali at SF General and was supposed to be a patient of yours once I was done with ABVD chemo (Hodgkin's lymphoma). At the time, both of you agreed—without a shred of doubt—that I should have a combination of chemotherapy and radiation treatment to ensure that I eradicate my disease, but now I'm told that's not the case from my new oncologist, Dr. Jaworski.

I know you're a renowned professional in your field, so I am confused why it has suddenly been decided that it would be best that I have 4 cycles of ABVD and no radiation treatment. When we met (I don't expect you to remember me), you even took the time to show me my PET scan to demonstrate that the mediastinal mass was large enough to merit the combination treatment.

I just need your reassurance that this sudden decision—to do ABVD treatment with no radiation treatment—*is what is in my best interest.*

When you have an opportunity, please, please give me a call to explain at (510) ***-****. I would really appreciate it.

Despite all this turmoil, I still met for lunch with my friend Andy. I was upset and flustered when he picked me up from my home. But thankfully for me, Andy is a rare man, a wonderful friend who actually seems to enjoy hearing other people's troubles. We became friends when we worked at a large nonprofit in San Francisco. He worked as a case manager for poor, elderly residents who needed in-home care due to their mental and/or physical disabilities. Once we became friends, Andy would take breaks to chill out in my cubicle in the Human Resources Department.

While we rode over to a Korean BBQ restaurant in Noe Valley, I was able to calm down a bit once I explained all the madness surrounding my treatment. As we ate our lunch, I received a call from an unknown San Francisco number. I apologized to Andy and excused myself. I stepped out to take the call.

"This is Juan," I said, looking down Castro Street.

"Hi Juan, Dr. Kirsch here," he said with a deliberate gusto, as if he were a plane traveling at its optimum cruising speed. "I received your message today. I have reviewed your file—including the PET scan that we took of you back in June. Before I explain to you why I think Dr. Jaworski is flat-out wrong in his assessment that you do not need radiation treatment or additional ABVD treatment, let me tell you that in all the years I have been in practice, it has been *very rare* that I have completely disagreed with a decision from a fellow practitioner. But in your case, I have to completely disagree with Dr. Jaworski— and the reason is because the cancerous mass in your mediastinal area *was* large enough to merit six cycles of ABVD treatment *and* radiation treatment."

I nodded as I slowly paced alongside the parked cars. Though it pained me to hear that I might have to continue chemotherapy, inside I was sighing in relief. It was intuitive, but I felt complete trust in this man.

"In all the years I've been in practice, I have never seen any studies that have shown that four cycles of ABVD treatment is sufficient to treat a Hodgkin's lymphoma patient like you, with the size that your mass was before you started chemotherapy. If Dr. Jaworski or Dr. Luce—his consulting oncologist—can produce findings that support such a treatment plan, then I can agree with his decision. [Dr. Luce was the director of Oncology Services at San Francisco General; she supervised all the oncology fellows during their practicum. Much later, I would learn that she oversaw any treatment decisions the fellows made for their patients.] But until then, I simply can't advise you to accept the treatment plan he has recommended for you."

"Okay," I said.

He went on to advise me not to take his medical opinion or Dr. Jaworski's alone. He suggested that I seek a second opinion from Stanford's excellent oncology faculty. This took me aback but in the best way. It wasn't like he was a salesman daring me to find a better deal elsewhere. His conviction was palpable, like something that breathed through my phone speaker. He did not stand to gain from my decision in any way. I could sense that he had only my best interests in mind, not some desire to be right.

Dr. Kirsch ended our call by assuring me that he would contact the oncology department at San Francisco General to sort out the matter. I thanked him for his swift response to my e-mail.

Walking back into the restaurant, I felt both relieved and deflated. The self-pity came soon afterward. I had to tell my family, friends, and classmates that the whole *I'm done with chemo!* was nothing but a big *psych.*

Seesaw

A WEEK AFTER we met at Socha Café, Paola and I went out on our first let's-see-how-this-goes date. We dined at a popular Burmese restaurant out in the Richmond District. It was a chilly night. I was dressed in a long-sleeve shirt, black pea coat, and some snazzy brown Oxfords I had just bought. Paola looked deliciously reportorial, as if she had come straight from work. However, her dress choice turned out to be fitting as our date had the feel of a job interview.

During our brief time apart, I had come to question whether Paola was the kind of woman I wanted to be in a relationship with. Once I reflected on my mother's birthday celebration, those murky feelings I had when Paola left, I realized that I also felt disappointed in that moment because I, ideally, wanted a girlfriend whose spirit was more like Tagi's instead of Paola's. And there were a number of things about Paola that I wasn't exactly hot about: her career choice, her appetite for swanky restaurants and nightlife spots (i.e., douchebag clubs, though she helped me to tolerate wine bars, which I consider a minor feat since I've always been a dive bar kind of guy), and her Catholic faith. Perhaps we were never right for each other? Perhaps what went down in Seattle was more of a self-destructive act on our relationship because I didn't have the guts to say, *This isn't quite working out*?

Once we sat down to eat, facing each other across our table, I grilled her. Why was she drawn to business journalism? (Though I always liked that she was a journalist, I had little respect for her profession in business journalism. Call me an idealist, but the only honorable journalists in my book are those who serve the public good.) What were her career goals? Did she think she would write more if she wasn't a

209

journalist? These were things I felt I should have known about her before. But I also asked these questions to assert a sense of power over our dating situation. To remind her that our date-to-date basis went both ways.

Paola told me that she liked the challenge that business journalism provided. She had worked for other newspapers where she had to cover boring events such as local dog shows and PTA meetings. Fluff pieces, she called them. Writing for a business journal was challenging because of the business entrepreneurs she had to interview. They were a driven, educated breed. Scheduling a lunch meeting or phone interview with them was an obstacle in itself. For her articles, Paola told me she liked uncovering details about a business deal, such as the revenue it was estimated to rake in or the exact square footage of a proposed building project. Her newspaper pieces were like puzzles she had to put together each week. And she enjoyed Thursday-morning meetings with the reporting staff where they pitched stories for the next paper.

As far as career, Paola told me she thought about someday becoming an editor. I was pleased to hear this. A month or so before, I had told her that perhaps she was more cut out to be an editor than a writer since she was proficient and incisive with her critiques for our writing group. (When I told her this, she pouted because she took it as a criticism of her lack of writing, which I didn't intend it to be.) I thought she could be a terrific editor—and it meant she wanted to work toward something. And as far as her creative writing, she was certain that she would get more done if she didn't sit in front of a computer at work most of the day.

Paola took these questions in stride. She didn't volley back with her own.

After dinner, we strolled over to Green Apple Books. We wandered about the maze of shelves, our shoes tapping loudly on the wooden floor. From time to time, we bumped into each other to show off a neat book we had happened upon.

Once I flicked through their calendars, searching for one for my dad, Paola and I reached out to hold hands. We smiled. Together, we winded through the store toward the register. While we did, I could feel my heart lull with ease.

In all likelihood, my relations with Paola's family took another mortal blow when her sister came to town a week later. Paola invited me and the other members of our writing group to the San Francisco Authors Luncheon, a fancy fundraiser at the downtown Hilton. Seats for the sold-out event went for $125 a pop. She had procured a few seats, free of cost, since her employer always reserved a table for the event.

The night before the luncheon, I sent Paola a text message. I can't remember what I wrote, but I think it was a sweet ditty—a good night, looking-forward-to-seeing-you-mañana kind of text. By the time I headed off to the Hilton the following morning, I had not received a response. And it really set me off. Maybe I'm old-fashioned, but I think it's rude to not respond to someone's e-mail, text, or phone call. To me, it's like walking down a street, greeting someone, and getting no response. It was completely unlike her not to respond. I presumed Paola was in preoccupied and distant mode like she tended to be when her family was in town.

But my response was a horrible, horrible overreaction.

After I signed in at the registration table, I made my way through the lavish ballroom to Paola's table. One of the authors was speaking at the podium to a packed house. Before I took a seat next to Scott, I gave a nonchalant wave to Paola. Her sister, Rosa, and roommate, Daisy, sat beside her. They were dressed as if it were a wedding reception.

For the next three hours, I proceeded to ignore Paola and her guests. Instead, I joked and conversed with Scott as though he was the only person at the table I knew. I even avoided making eye contact with Paola. My rationale was that things were clearly not improving between us, so why should I bother being chatty to people who were not going to be a part of my life?

At the time, thanks to a lightened class load, I was devouring Thich Nhat Hanh's *Anger: Wisdom for Cooling the Flames*. He's a Buddhist monk who has written a ton of books on Buddhism, peace, and love. One of his first teachings that struck me was when he explained that anger stemmed from suffering. That was so simple to understand, yet I had never made that connection. He also wrote about how to use "loving language" with loved ones in order to communicate one's anger in a constructive way.

So clearly, Nhat Hanh's teachings were having little to no immediate impact on my behavior then. As much as I sincerely desired to be a better partner for Paolita, reading that book was just a first step toward making *any* positive change. And his book didn't warn me about the perils of making assumptions. Like the ones I made about the text Paola didn't respond to.

Once the luncheon was over, I spoke for a few minutes with Rosa. On my way out, I curtly said good-bye to Paola, thanked her for inviting me, though there was zero gratitude in my voice. When she asked if I wanted any of the hardcover books of the authors who were on the panel—complementary gifts given to her employer—I said, "No thanks." She was flustered by my cold, standoffish behavior. (I can still see and feel the confusion in her pleading eyes. And it tears at me now, though it didn't then.)

Paola sent a text later that day. She asked why I ignored her at the luncheon. I told her I felt sour toward her because she ignored the text I had sent her.

She told me she never received it.

At first, I was doubtful. This had never happened before. My cell phone didn't respond with a "failed to send" message. But I believed her because she was always honest with me.

I apologized for the misunderstanding. Paola and I got over it because she was incredibly forgiving of me. But I must have made yet another unfavorable impression on her family. The twenty-first-century telltale sign? Paola's friend Daisy unfriended me on Facebook shortly after the luncheon.

Halloween

A WEEK AFTER my ninth infusion, I stood at Justin Herman Plaza in front of the majestic Ferry Building among hundreds of other cyclists. The sun was setting over the city's skyline. The unmistakable scent of marijuana perfumed the air. It was Critical Mass's Halloween ride. (Critical Mass was a monthly happening in which cyclists gathered to pedal through the city like a centipede of bicycles. It was started in San Francisco as a way of promoting cycling as a sexy, non-gas-guzzling means of transportation.) I was dressed up again in my Catholic school-girl outfit. My friend Judy stood beside me. She looked cute in a Trojan soldier outfit she made herself—a black plastic helmet and chest armor made of cardboard, plastic, and tape. It was her idea to join the ride. The Halloween ride was a spectacle, always a bit extra kooky and impassioned since many of the bicyclists dressed up for it.

Once our two-wheel parade got underway, Judy and I pedaled down Market Street at a turtle's pace. We were amid a bottleneck of bicyclists siphoning out into downtown. We gawked and laughed and pointed at the costumes we dug: a guy dressed up in a full-body Scooby Doo suit, the Cookie Monster, Pee Wee Herman, a guy dressed in a feathered chicken outfit. There was also a family of ghosts, hordes of pirates, and a trio of rapscallion Santas weaving and darting through the mass of cyclists on BMX bikes. Many of us gyrated to the electronic dance music that pulsed from the large speakers a few cyclists lugged.

The highlight of the ride was when we rode through the Broadway Tunnel. When we approached the two-lane tunnel with dull-yellow walls, I whipped out the voice recorder I had packed in the tiny blue clutch that hung from my handlebar. Cycling with one hand, I began recording. I was near the front of the mass, having separated from Judy shortly after the ride commenced. As the first bicyclists entered the tunnel, I screamed "QUIET!" since there was a sign at the beginning of the tunnel's walkway that urges pedestrians to keep the noise down. A few bicyclists chortled, then started yelling *wooooooooooooooo!* with me as we clogged up the tunnel—our shouts, elated hoots, and ringing bells fusing into one glorious roaring echo that washed over us as we zipped through the tunnel. It had been nearly a year since I had cycled in Critical Mass, since I had screamed my head off in either the Broadway or Stockton Tunnel. I didn't think I was going to die anytime soon, but I had already learned that such things couldn't be taken for granted. So I hooted and barked (yeah, barked) and shrieked with all my being, with complete glee for that moment we had been blessed with.

Later that night, I strolled out of the Glen Park station with a large paper bag and girly clutch in hand. My schoolgirl outfit was complemented with a fantastic dirty-blonde bob wig I had borrowed from Judy that screamed cheap hooker. I strolled past the freeway underpass into the Excelsior neighborhood. Once I ascended a stairwell alit in orange streetlight to Mission Street, I felt a flood of nostalgia come over me. Three years before, I used to regularly cycle down that hill into the Excelsior to be with my heartachingly beautiful half-Chilean girlfriend, Julia. She was the ex-girlfriend whose car I vandalized in a fit of rage on my twenty-seventh birthday (which, to this day, is still the one act in my life I regret the most). But before that horrible end, I had loved her like no one before her. We had our share of contented, loving moments during the eleven months we were together. (The Excelsior hillside at night always reminds me of Julia. I can still remember how twinkly and picturesque the houses on the often-misty hillside looked from her bedroom, like we were in the midst of a constellation that was not a part of this world.) A month after I met Julia, I told my best friend that I thought she was "the one"—that someday she would be the mother of my children. It was a ridiculously bold proclamation to make, but I believed it (though, of course, it starkly illuminated the naïveté and sense of abandon I had then about matters of love).

And so, as I made my way down Mission Street to the Halloween party, I became filled with a sense of longing and regret.

At the front door of my former coworker's house, I could hear throbbing dance music and a droning chatter. I took a breath before I waltzed in with a bottle of red wine and a six-pack in the bag. The odds were highly favorable for an interesting night. And an emotional one, too. I had not seen many of my former coworkers since I left to attend grad school over a year earlier (i.e., Life before Lymphoma). I was going to see Bryan, who was one of the party DJs. He was the only colleague at the party who knew I had lymphoma. Before I began treatment, he helped me to see chemotherapy in a more positive light—as something that would ultimately heal me. And I would assuredly see several of the case managers with whom I used to drink and shoot the shit after work, including Caitlin, whom I used to be crazy for. I was nervous and excited at the prospect of seeing her, of revisiting a second love in one night.

And sure enough, I saw my old peeps. Standing in a crowded kitchen teeming with finger foods and bottles of alcohol, we caught up. We talked about how grad school was working out for me, about their work, and how things had changed at the nonprofit they still worked at since I left. It was all light and fun. Whenever any one of them said, "Hey Juan! How are you doing?" or "Whatcha been up to?" my initial thought was, *Well, I recently got diagnosed with a rare cancer. . . . But, anyway, how 'bout you?* I treated such questions like an expert mata-dor, flourishingly sidestepping that Debbie Downer of Debbie Downers (¡olé!) by saying, "Nothing much! Just working part time and going to grad school." (If I may gloat, it was a clever response because they could inquire about either of those two facets of my life. Or, I could go on and talk about how utterly fascinating the transition from full-time tool to grad student was for me.)

I did feel disingenuous responding like that, though.

Like a bit of a liar.

But the alternative—dropping the cancer bomb unsuspectingly at a Halloween party (insert deafening roar of an atomic bomb exploding here)—was *not* a choice.

As the night motored along, I moseyed over to the makeshift dance floor (i.e., the living room) with a half-empty bottle of wine in hand. Bryan manned the DJ stand. Ironically, Bryan was dressed in a black grim reaper robe. Beside the turntables lay a comical mask of our gov-ernator, Arnold Schwarzenegger. (Bryan put it on later, which gave him a refreshingly disturbing appearance.) He stepped around to give me a hug. He told me he was glad I came out, that I looked great. He asked how I was. I truthfully told him I felt fine. I explained that my last infusion had been a week before, that the first few days after the infusion were, thankfully, the only time I felt weak. Then he introduced me to his wife, Julia. She was also dressed in a ghoulish black robe. Her face and hands were painted in a devilish red that looked phosphorous. It made her look toxic, which made me think about the cytotoxins flowing through my insides.

After I danced and conversed with Julia about her homeland of Russia, I excused myself. I boogied into the kitchen. I took another slug from the bottle, then giggled when I dribbled a splotch on my blouse. The room was a busy hive of chatter. I got caught up in a delirious and raunchy conversation with some ex-coworkers and two flamboyant gay men who worked with them. One of them went uh-uh, no-no, you-need-to-make-your-outfit-more-trashy on me. I stood in their mini-circle while the flirty, hilarious guy knotted the bottom of my blouse, jailbait-style, to expose my hairy paunch. We all roared. Then I saw Caitlin standing a little off by herself beside a counter littered with bottles of booze and red party cups that had been forsaken. Her boyfriend and coworkers were not around.

Her eyes lit up when I stepped over to her. She was dressed in a goofy homemade bedbug outfit. (Earlier in the evening, I gave her props on her getup, which she was all too elated to tell me was an inside joke since many of her clients had bedbugs in their homes.) I asked how her crazy clients were before I started in with the conversation I had really hoped this night would produce.

"Hey, remember that swollen lymph node I had last year?" I asked, my voice a tad slurry.

"Yeah—" Caitlin said, an uncomfortable smile surfacing.

"Well, it turns out I had cancer after all. Hodgkin's lymphoma—a pretty rare blood cancer. I wanted to tell you, not because I was dying to tell you some bad news but because you were there for me from the very beginning."

She nodded, then rubbed the side of my arm.

"But I don't want you to feel sad. It's not entirely bad news. I think it's going to make me a better person. And it's really treatable, so my odds of surviving—at least this time around—are good. I'm getting ABVD—four different kinds of chemo. I'm halfway through my fifth cycle. I get it every two weeks over at San Francisco General."

We stood there silently after my mouth went cancer-potty on her. I rattled off all those details because Caitlin was familiar with cancer. Her mom—a lifelong smoker and recovering alcoholic—had already undergone two bouts of breast cancer.

"But that *is* bad news," Caitlin said. "All you've had to go through—and still have to."

"Well, yeah. Pffftt, it *is* fucked up, but what can I do?" I asked, throwing my hands up for punctuation.

Then I snickered.

"You know what's funny? That Susan G. Komen race we ran? I *had* cancer then. I should've been wearing a pink shirt. I just didn't know it."

Though it was a morose conversation, it felt good to finally share these things with Caitlin. When I was diagnosed, she was one of the first people I wanted to tell. But after we stopped working together, after I decided that we shouldn't continue to see each other behind her boyfriend's back, she didn't want to stay in touch. I think it was easier for her. For a short while, her absence left me heartbroken. I missed her sardonic humor. Her tomboy spirit. Her kiddie smile. Her midwestern inflection when she said words that made me smile like "douchebag," "crabby pants," or "for Chrissakes!"

Some of her coworkers eventually stepped in from the porch. Caitlin and I started up conversations with them and went our separate ways again.

I had brought that bottle of wine with the hopes of drinking nothing else, but once I was tipsy, I stayed at the party far longer than I anticipated. I started in on the shitty keg beer out on the porch, then tag-teamed it with some whisky. And before I knew it, I reached the level of sloppy drunkenness where I just keep going, where I am liable to drink until I puke or pass out.

After many of the revelers left the party, I made my way to the dance floor. Numb, drunk, and a smidge sad, I danced alone, closing my eyes in my attempt to establish some form of harmony between the mesh of emotions swirling within me and the pulsing music and twirling party lights, this bizarre reality that was the script I was the active protagonist of. At one point, I opened my eyes—probably to make sure that I didn't stumble into one of the speakers. I saw Caitlin standing in the kitchen doorway. She was watching over me. It was a flash, but her face had a solemn expression before she turned back into the kitchen.

An hour or so later, my drunk ass boarded one of the all-night buses on Mission Street. I had untied my blouse to cover my paunch, but I was still rocking the cheap-floosie wig. When I took a seat near the front, I could hear the noise level in the bus drop. I could feel eyes on me. Probably a few of the homies who lived in the east side of the Mission. They might have thought I was a fag, un maricón, as they would say. And so, I spread my legs out in a very unladylike fashion while I leaned back in my seat like I could not give one fuck about anything. I might as well have held out my arms and barked, "What? What?—putos" at them all. That could've been fun.

Made Me Nuclear

AT 6:20 P.M., while sitting in the semicircle of tables in my workshop class, my phone alarm sounded. Our class was critiquing the last manuscript of the day. As quietly as I could, I stood and slung my backpack on, clutched my helmet against my hip, and tiptoed past my classmates. It was the first time I had ever left any of my graduate classes early. It felt wrong to leave, especially our workshop class, but I had a play to catch in the city.

Once I snapped the front and taillights onto Blue, then put on my gloves, helmet, sweater, and headphones, the time on my cell phone read 18:23. I had ample time to catch the 6:55 p.m. train to San Francisco. The nighttime ride through the pitch-dark hillside to the Lafayette station usually took me twenty minutes.

On my way down a steep hill, my bicycle rolled over some uneven pavement. My front light dislodged and bounced off into the gravel that lined the trail. I had forgotten that the light had slipped off my bike a few days before; the part that snapped into the base had broken. Since I was rolling down the hill at a speed of at least twenty miles per hour, I came to a halt fifteen feet away. The front light was swallowed by the dark. There were no lights in that wooded hillside. I detached the taillight and walked back to where the light must have fallen. I shined the red light on the gravel and found the front light and its battery cover, but the batteries had bounced off somewhere.

Shit.

I took my iPod out of my butt pocket and pointed its luminescent light and the red taillight all over the gravel. Still no sign of the batteries.

I looked at the time on my iPod.

I had twenty-eight minutes to catch the train.

The musical I had left class early for was *Made Me Nuclear*. It was a one-time performance at the Marsh, a small theater two blocks from my home. Though I normally abhorred musicals—too disturbingly cheerful for my taste (unless they were dark and twisted like *Chicago*, *Little Shop of Horrors*, or *Sweeney Todd: The Demon Barber of Fleet Street*)—this one was a must-see. It was a solo show written and performed by Charlie Lustman, a middle-aged musician who had developed an exceptionally rare form of cancer. The play was a musical odyssey of his cancer journey. I had to see how he expressed his story, how he evoked the emotions I was going through and now trying to translate into words.

I could not waste any more time trying to find the batteries. I grabbed my bike and jogged up the shadowy hillside toward the road. Though winding and perilous since it was narrow with little shoulder room, the road at least had streetlights.

But once I cycled past a pool of orange streetlight, I was back in pitch dark. I stared down at the pavement in front of me. I could hardly make out the vague, milky-white line that marked the shoulder of the road. To my sides were rock outcrops. Large rocks and gravel littered the ground. The shoulder of the road was no more than two feet wide. I was frightened—scared of hitting an unseen bump and falling onto the road. Scared of getting hit from behind by a car that failed to see me in time. Gripping the handlebars tightly, I pedaled along the faint line as best as I could.

A pair of glaring headlights shot through the blanket of darkness in the opposite direction. When they approached, the headlights blinded me. Once the vehicle passed, I heard another one behind me. I pedaled as far out on the narrow shoulder of the road as I could. My heart was thumping. The car swung around me. Their front and taillights briefly illuminated the road ahead. I pedaled as hard as I could after seeing that the road was smooth and free of bumps, rocks, and potholes. Another car soon followed. Again, I rode their coattail of light. Like this, I covered the half-mile of dark winding road until I rolled into a residential area alit with streetlights. Flashing a cocksure smirk à la Indiana Jones, I pedaled on with gusto.

Once I walked into the Marsh, I became a little nervous. And cancer-paranoid. There were a handful of people in the small theater—mostly middle-aged white folks. Predominantly couples. Like 4C, I was without question the youngest person there. I sat by myself near the middle of the seating area, a few rows from the stage. I felt naked. Outed. Assuredly, the people there could tell I had cancer. Why else would I have a cropped head in the beginning of November? And why else would I be seeing *this* play?

Thankfully, I had the program to bury my attention into. Before long, the theater owner stepped onto the stage to thank us for coming. The show's producer—who had come all the way from Santa Monica—had some moving words about his involvement in the play before Charlie Lustman took the stage.

A youthful-looking man in his early forties, Charlie came out donning sunglasses and a shiny white suit that appeared fit for space travel. A radiation warning sign was stitched onto the center of his chest. His bald head looked like it had been buffed at a bowling alley. His sunglasses brimmed beneath the lone spotlight that he stepped into. He kind of resembled guitar virtuoso Joe Satriani—except when it came to their instruments. Strapped around his shoulder was an acoustic guitar that had been given a rainbow-groovy finish, as though he had stepped back to the Summer of Love and stolen it from some free-love hippie at a Jefferson Airplane concert in Golden Gate Park (*Hey man, that's my ax!*). A microphone headset hung over one of his ears. He waved at us before he began to play his opening song.

For his first tune, Charlie sung about waiting for that dreaded phone call from his doctor. A telephone rang, then he acted out receiving it—his version of the Bad News. Once the song took its morose course, he walked over to a keyboard. He played and sung his story. I related with him from the get-go. While I sat there, his song set off an explosion of synapses, a medley of sensations and memories. I remembered when I used to get choked up at the idea of receiving such a dreaded call while at school, work, or while walking around my neighborhood. The possibility of *that* phone call was like walking around with a bomb that could set off anywhere.

After he finished the first number to a round of applause, Charlie turned a wooden chair so that its back faced the audience. Straddling the chair, he began to tell us what must have been a scripted and rehearsed monologue but felt like an intimate, spontaneous conversation. Charlie began by telling us that he had just turned forty when he was diagnosed. He had just sold a theater that he had successfully run for years in Los Angeles—the only movie house in the country that exclusively screened silent films. He did so in order to devote himself to his music. And his wife was expecting their second child. It was supposed to be a glorious time in his life—until his dentist noticed a lump on his jaw during a standard cleaning. The dentist had no idea what it was. Soon after, Charlie was diagnosed with osteosarcoma—a form of bone cancer that is diagnosed among a handful of people each year in the United States. Any of us had better odds of winning the lottery *twice* in our lifetimes than developing that cancer, he told us. Since it was on his jaw, the doctors would have to saw it off and then replace it with a prosthetic mouthpiece that they would nail and fuse with his remaining jawbone. (They ended up removing three-quarters of his jaw.) On top of that, Charlie had to undergo radiation treatment in the basement of the same hospital where, a few floors up, his wife would give birth to their second child.

I was absolutely floored by his story. Staring at him—watching his mouth open and close to talk to us—was mind-blowing. I felt like I had stumbled upon an extraordinary moment.

Charlie went on to sing a total of twelve tunes that chronicled his insane journey. He sung a goofy yet emotional song about chemo brain, which made me laugh a bunch. He hopped back on the keyboard to play a somber song about how there were times he just wanted to give up while being sequestered in the hospital, which disallowed him from going out in public, let alone seeing his newborn daughter (which must have been heartbreaking). He wrote a George Harrison–Beatlesque-maharishi song with sitars about the newfound spirituality he developed while he struggled for his life. He ended with a cheerful ditty in which he sung about how simple life had become for him. His mantra: do what you love all the time.

The twenty-four audience members stood and applauded him for a long, long time. He smiled and blew kisses to us. A few audience members stepped onstage to talk to him and his manager. I was tempted to walk over to him to begin to tell him what his performance, what the work he was doing meant to me. (Before performing in San Francisco he played at a pediatric hospital in Seattle that treated children with leukemia.) But I figured it would have been verbal diarrhea—a manic rant about how glorious I thought he was. So instead I bought his CD and left, telling myself that it would be best to send him an eloquent, heartfelt e-mail in which I could form my thoughts in a more coherent way besides, *Oh my gosh, oh my gosh, oh my gosh! You were IMMAC-ULATE!*

On my stroll home with Blue, I buzzed from the mix of thoughts and emotions Charlie's performance had stirred within me. I don't think I have ever felt like that in my life: inspired, mesmerized, moved, validated, humbled, and nourished in the most profound way. I felt light with utter glee—like an effulgent balloon that could float to the near-full moon. I felt so inspired by the beauty he had managed to create from his ordeal, humbled by how he had given himself to us through his musical. It made me feel like I was on the right path—that I, too, could come out of my trying time a better, more loving person. And I was validated in my belief that I should pour myself, my being, into a work to share with others.

In one night, Charlie Lustman rocketed to the top among all the men and women I clutched to my heart and called my heroes.

Peeling

MY TENTH INFUSION was the first one that fucked me up. First one that made me think, *Now* this *is what chemo is supposed to be like.* Sunday morning, two days after round ten, I awoke with a particularly bad fit of chemo coughing. I whipped up a hearty breakfast in hopes of bringing it to a halt. After I ate, I sat at my desk and flicked a piece of paper that bounced off my recycling basket. When I leaned over to grab it, I felt the need to cough. Breakfast came out instead, splattering in and around my trash can. An accidental barfing. This had happened a few times. For the rest of the day, I felt grody—as though my pores were emitting nauseous toxic exhaust. Like I was a walking Chemo-Potty. The anti-nausea medication could not banish that nasty feeling away.

A couple of days later, my right arm began to hurt. It burned like my left arm did after my first infusion, though the pain was not as sharp. By then, both of my arms had each received five infusions. And it showed. The veins on my right arm were dark and tough like cords when I ran my fingers over them. And so, even though I didn't want to, I drank a bottle of red wine for the next two nights to numb the pain. I reasoned that it was safer than popping pills such as Advil, which the oncology staff discouraged me from taking since it could induce stomach bleeding.

Around that time, I became fixated on snakes. I've loved them since I was a kid. (The first pet I ever wanted was a ball python, but my parents talked me out of it.) My thirty-year-old, chemo-infused self was fascinated that a number of ancient cultures had revered them. The Mayans esteemed snakes because they could shed their skins, as though they could transform themselves. I wanted to shed myself of the destructive thoughts and habits I had developed during my adulthood. I felt like any long-term survival depended on this change.

Wow . . .

THOUGH SHE WAS out of town for four weekends in late October and November, opening a chapter of her Latina sorority at a small university in Eastern Washington, Paola and I continued to go out. I bought a bouquet of flowers and had them delivered to her office. She sent a text saying, "Thanks for the flowers! What a surprise! You really didn't have to do this." But I *did* feel like I had to do such an act. I needed to prove to her, and myself, that I could be the sweeter guy she believed I could be.

Around that time, Paola told me something that has stuck with me. We were in her bedroom, standing near her bed. The morning fog had lifted. The sun shined through the window blinds. I was complaining about something; I can't remember what. Paola responded by saying, "You know, the entire time I've known you, I don't think I've seen you really happy."

My jaw dropped.

"Paola, I have *cancer*," I said. "I've been battling it half of this year. Not exactly the best time to be cheery about life."

"I know, but still. I've talked to my family about it, and they say that's still not an excuse to be unhappy. There are always rough patches in life."

Now that I look back on that time, I am stunned that I didn't respond with a wide-eyed "WOW" and bolt. Instead, I said, "Well, I think battling cancer is a pretty exceptional circumstance. It doesn't happen to everyone. And none of you can understand what it's like because you haven't had to go through it."

We were silent. Then Paola told me, like she had on prior occasions, that I tended to have a pessimistic outlook on life. Focused a bit too much on the negative instead of the positive in life. She did have a point, but still. How could she have said such a thing? And so cavalierly? Even then, a meek voice inside of me whispered these thoughts. It was only much, much later when this memory resurfaced and my retrospective interior narrator boomed those questions.

But because I still desperately believed in our relationship, because I was trying to atone for all the times I had fucked up, I stayed in her room. I pushed down what she said. I was blind to what it meant.

When the Gaels Got Outhustled

WITH NINE SECONDS left in the basketball game, Paola and I stood with the raucous capacity crowd at McKeon Pavilion. Saint Mary's had the ball and was down by two to twenty-fourth-ranked Vanderbilt. Paola proudly donned a navy-blue shirt of her alma mater. Our seats were in the front row in a second-tier section with a few of the other Commodore fans in attendance. I stood against the railing, pogoing with excitement. I pointed my voice recorder toward the court, toward the mass of undergraduates in front of me who had cheered on our team all game long. Eight hours before, I had wobbled out of 4C. I was down to my last infusion.

"C'mon, baby, c'mon!" I shouted as the Gaels inbounded from Vanderbilt's end. My voice was hoarse. During the second half, I had shouted with abandon when Saint Mary's roared back from a crowd-silencing 57–43 deficit.

Our outstanding freshmen guard, Matthew Dellavedova, got the ball. He dribbled it up court. Once he passed the half-court line, he flung the ball to a streaking Steindl, a 6'7" forward with three-point range. Steindl was well-defended, so he frantically dribbled to the corner. He pump-faked his defender off. He had an open look! The crowd gasped as he spotted up for a game-winning three, the final seconds ticking off. It all seemed to happen so fast—my mouth dropping as we saw the ball rainbow toward the basket (*Oh my god, oh my god, WE'RE GONNA WIN!*), then watched it clang off the rim, the crowd groaning in defeat as the buzzer sounded.

"Oh, man!" I said, hitting the stop button on my voice recorder. Paola was beaming. I was happy her team had won, super happy she had suggested we attend the game, and grateful that I was able to make it. I was a bit surprised that I was able to muster up the energy I had. The long nap after my infusion helped. Even more surprising was that I somehow felt better after my eleventh infusion than my tenth. I am certain it was due to the acupuncture I received a day before. Amber had recommended her acupuncturist, Robert—a man she considered a healer. I was proud of myself for seeking his help. My precancer self would have considered such a visit an indulgence, something I didn't *need*, but I was learning to give more love to the vessel I was fortunate to have.

"Wow, what a game," Paola said, as everybody in the gym began to file out.

Smiling, I rubbed her shoulder.

"Yeah, man, I think that's the most exciting sports game I've ever seen in person."

Paola put her hands on her hips and gave me a reproachful look.

"Hey, don't call me *man!*" she said playfully.

"I'm sorry," I said, pouting my lips, dramatically hanging my head before I broke into a grin.

I knew I probably shouldn't have gone to the game—an event with a crowd of germ-carrying humans—while my immune system was depleted. But one of my main strategies in ridding my body of lymphoma was to go about life as normally as possible without being flat-out delusional of my physical capabilities. I thought it was good for my spirit to partake in activities that made me happy—a strategy I picked up from Norman Cousins's book. Plus, I was determined to make it my final school year, so I wasn't about to miss that game with Paolita.

We shuffled along with the herd of people exiting the gym. Once outside, Paola and I held hands all the way to her car, feeling full and victorious.

My Cancer Reading

MOM AND DAD sat to my left as we watched Isaac, one of my beloved classmates, a fellow nutball who sported a long beard that made him look like a ZZ Top apprentice, finish reading a short story. Four other second-year classmates had already gone up to the podium to read in front of the crowd gathered at the Soda Center. The room was packed— about seventy to eighty people in attendance. Our longtime family friend, Señora Coty, sat beside my parents. Paola sat behind us since she showed up halfway through the reading after a long day at work. A few other friends were in the audience. I was reading last. It had been a night I had looked forward to since the beginning of the semester. In the e-mail invitation I sent out weeks before, I wrote, "I'll have to be hospitalized or seriously ill to miss this reading."

The crowd applauded when Isaac finished. Then Xochitl, my friend and classmate, stepped up to the podium to introduce me. With my manuscripts sitting on my lap, my hands folded over them, I stared at my feet as she said some tenderhearted things about me. Before I knew it, she was saying, "And without further ado, my friend, Juan Alvarado Valdivia."

"Here we go," I said to my parents, the crowd applauding while I wiggled out of our row.

"Wow, thank you, Xochitl. That was too kind," I said at the podium, my hand over my heart as I looked out to her. "Can we just leave after that? I mean, I don't know if I can follow that up!"

This made Xochitl laugh as well as others in the crowd. After I straightened my papers in a neat pile, I looked out over the crowd. I took in the view from behind the podium.

"I wanna—thank you all for being here," I said, nearly stammering. "I'm really grateful to be able to read to you."

Since the day before, I had imagined that moment—thought of what I wanted and *needed* to share with the audience. But once I stood up there, it was difficult to remember what I had practiced. Everything seemed a little too fast, like I was swept up in a powerful current with no pause button. My thoughts and emotions felt like a bunch of bouncing balls in an empty room. I looked at Skye, one of my classmates, who sat in front of me. She had an empathetic expression. I think she could sense how much it meant for me to be there.

"Before I begin, there's one thing you need to know for my reading, although many of you already know: I was recently diagnosed with Hodgkin's lymphoma. But I don't want you to feel sad. Don't want you to feel boo-hoo-hooey for me. Thankfully, it's a really treatable cancer, and so far the treatment's been really effective."

The crowd broke into applause. I bent my head and giggled and thanked them.

"Before I start, and I apologize, because I know I've probably already gone over my time, I want to thank my classmates, especially my non-fiction classmates for all the help you've given me to become a better writer. I want to thank my professors, especially my mentors Wesley and Marilyn. I want to thank my friends and family for coming all the way out here to Moraga. I really appreciate it. I want to dedicate this reading to all of you but especially to my parents, because none of this would have been possible without all the love and support you've always given to me."

I looked at my parents when I said that. I could hear the crowd applaud as I saw my mom get emotional.

"So this is my cancer reading. I'm gonna read three short pieces from my memoir. This first one is called "Quién Sabe, or Who Knows.""[*]

To my complete surprise, a few people tittered while I rattled off the various theories I had concocted as to the cause of my disease. I think it made them nervous—as though they realized that this could also happen to them or their loved ones. I looked out into the crowd and ad-libbed, "Yeah, it really crossed my mind!" after I read about the whole chewing-my-toenails bit. It got the crowd laughing.

[*] This was an earlier incarnation of "Why? (The Inevitable Why)."

My mom held up her camera to snap a picture of me. By the time I got to the part where I wrote that she thought cancer must have been "a test from God," I could see she was crying. Part of me felt saddened (what son wants to make his mother cry?), but I relished the opportunity to look at her while I read that paragraph so she could hear my truth, my rejection of her God. This was nothing new between us. Over the years, we have had a few spirited tiffs over our spiritual differences, but like any great mother, she has always accepted me. (Mom accompanied me to the Thrift Town in Fremont when I shopped for my Catholic schoolgirl outfit. I asked for her opinion when I tried on a sultry red dress that didn't quite fit. Why, she was the one who picked out my blouse and cute black slippers!) But it *was* something to read that section aloud to her. It got my heart drumming.

I continued on with an early chapter that I eventually cut. Before long, it was time to read my final piece, "Someday You'll Be Sorry"—a piece my nonfiction classmates loved. I told the audience that the piece was based on an old Louis Armstrong song I became enchanted with after I was diagnosed. Then I apologized to everyone because I was going to sing parts of the song.

While I read the opening description of the ballroom, I looked out into the crowd to make eye contact with them. *I had them.* They were following every word I said. Inside, I was delirious with joy. When I got to the part when my character sings the tune into Mr. Hodgkins's ears, I nodded rhythmically to replicate the song's swingy rhythm. Then I sung those lyrics in a jazzy, pseudo-Armstrong voice that could not have been pleasing to the ear. But it made me smile, so I went with it. The crowd seemed to dig it, too. I said "thank you" once I finished.

The crowd clapped as I walked back to my parents. I felt like a proud kid who had just won a spelling bee. Once I took my seat, I turned to my mom and patted her thigh.

"Te quiero mucho, mochito," she said.

"Yo también," I said, then leaned forward to smile at my dad. My professor, Marilyn, grinned as she stepped behind the podium.

"Thank you to all our readers," she said. "I think that was the best student reading we have ever had. Thank you all for coming!"

We all stood, the room bursting with chatter.

The next five or ten minutes was congratulatory bedlam. Señora Coty rubbed my back and told me I did a great job. My friend Risa—who I have jokingly called "the Jewish grandmother I never had"—was the first of my classmates to come over to hug and congratulate me. I embraced and profusely thanked my friend Amber for driving from way the fuck out in the Sunset District to catch my reading, then chitchatted with my friend Judy Johnson-Williams—the teaching artist for the K–5 arts education program I wrote grants for. Paolita gave me a congratulatory hug, too.

Once my parents bid me good night, Wesley came over to hug me. A rumor was zigzagging around the room that many of the students were heading over to the Roundup Saloon for postreading libations. Wesley asked if he could hitch a ride with us.

We rode up to the Roundup just as many of my classmates were arriving. A number of first-year students who I was not familiar with congratulated me on my reading. It made me feel like I had won a beauty pageant or something.

It was festive inside the divey bar. Twenty or so of my classmates were there, including my old classmate Barbara and her husband. She told me how much she liked my new material—how my writing had improved since the previous school year. I thanked her. It felt good to hear. It helped to affirm that I was on the right path—that this was the book I was born to write.

My peeps were splintered off in their circles throughout the bar. I swirled about, joining a conversation here, catching a snippet there. Being the cool-ass professor he was, Wesley drank and hobnobbed with us. (On the ride over to the bar, Wesley—tee-hee drunk from the wine served at the reception before the reading—told us a dirty Santa joke his sister had taught him.[*] He acted out a seemingly innocent exchange between a little girl sitting on Santa's lap that ended with her saying, "Because your finger smells like pussy," which made us roar.) Like a jolly bee, I buzzed about the bar, congratulating my peeps on their readings. I made a toast with the guys from my program I was especially fond of. Our time together was fleeting. We had a semester left before graduating.

---

[*] After I submitted the first chapters of this memoir to our writing workshop, Wesley told me about his sister when we rode a train back into the city. A few years before, she had cancer. He hung out with her a lot while she underwent chemotherapy. He loved to tell me that one of the first things she asked her oncologist was if she could continue to drink wine during treatment. And he told me that she made it through.

Wesley told me all this to comfort me—and to show that he was not afraid to converse about cancer. The rest of my Saint Mary's community was supportive in much the same way, bless them.

About an hour after we stepped into the Roundup, Wesley and I huddled together. We were standing against the bar.

"I am *wasted*," he said to me in confidence.

I busted up and gave him a hearty pat on the shoulder.

"All right, bye, my dear," he said. "You were great."

We leaned in for a hug good-bye. While we embraced, Wesley surprised me by giving me a big smooch on my cheek. I could feel my smile blossom even further. Probably blushed with Santa-like cheeks. Leaning back against the counter, I watched him walk past the crowd and out the saloon doors. I turned to face the bar for a few seconds to bask in the moment I had been graced with, the affection he had given. Forget Chuck Palahniuk when he rightly wrote in *Fight Club*, "You are not special. You're not a beautiful and unique snowflake." I felt pretty damn special then.

Call it wishful thinking, but that night I felt like I was firmly grounded on my long journey toward becoming like Wesley someday—a man immersed and devoted to writing. Someday, I hope to nurture and arm my own posse of budding writers. (I like to think of a successful creative writing program as a mini-Hogwarts of sorts. For word wizardry, of course.) I want to help others sing and roar the spirits within them. I want to give back what I have been fortunate enough to learn.

Besides being alive and healthy, there is not much more I want than to be a keeper of that sacred flame.

The Final Round

ON MY CALENDAR, December 4 was marked: "Chemo #12—the last one!"

That day had come.

As usual, I left the house with Metallica's "Of Wolf and Man" blaring from my headphones. The morning sun had lifted above the Victorians on tranquil Fair Oaks Street. Birds chirped in the trees. Kids stepped out of their houses with their mothers following behind. While I walked up the hill to the bus stop on 24th Street, my feet didn't have the determined bounce, the "I'm gonna fuck you up, Hodgkins" gusto that they had for the previous infusions. I was tired of that dance. I was going the full twelve rounds. I thought I had fought well. The day before I had cycled to and from school, something I never thought my body would have been capable of before I began treatment. I never missed a class during the fall semester. But I was done. Done fighting. Done pushing myself. Done putting on a game face every two weeks, lacing up those imaginary gloves on my way to 4C where I would sit on a chair and rest my arm, clench my hand into a fist—hungry to live, ravenous for rebirth—and stare ahead as though I was toe to toe with Mr. Hodgkins.

Two hours later, I was zonked out from the Benadryl and Ativan. I sat on a reclining chair that faced the doors into the infusion room. An IV was pricked into my right forearm, the inflatable cuff of a blood pressure monitor strapped around my left bicep. Vilma gently nudged my arm. "Juan," she said. I startled awake and saw her standing beside me.

"You have to sign off on the authorization," she said with her Filipina accent. She held out a clipboard and pen. "Just sign right there."

Barely able to keep my eyes half-open, I signed off on the release.

"Thank you," she said, taking them back. A woozy glimmer of glee surfaced within me. It was the last authorization I would have to sign. No more infusions to schedule. As she scribbled something into my file, I jolted in my chair after I remembered the card I had brought.

"Vilma," I said, "before I forget, I have a thank-you card for you and the nurses."

Turning her head to the side, she smiled in a you-shouldn't-have way.

"Oh, thank you, Juan," she said as I handed her the card. She held the white envelope up and said, "Nurses! Nurses, we got a card."

Vilma walked out of the infusion room toward the nurse's lounge. I fell back asleep.

An hour and a half later, I woke to find Vilma sitting on the stool beside me. She wore a medical mask that covered her nose and mouth. The inflatable cuff over my left bicep inflated tightly as it automatically did throughout my infusion to ensure that my blood pressure was not at a dangerous level. She was attaching one of the chemo push syringes into my IV.

"All right, Juan," Vilma said. "Your last one."

I peered down at the syringe, at the clear liquid being pushed into my bloodstream. I managed a grin because I felt I should for the Last One.

My parents were not standing against the wall like they had throughout my other infusions—including round eleven, in which I handed them my digital camera to take pictures of me during my infusion. (I wanted cancer mementos. Photographic documentation of a perilous juncture in my life, a place I did not wish to physically revisit.) They weren't even in the same area code. At that moment, they were somewhere in Cabo San Lucas of all places. My mom—who didn't even like to go out to eat because she thought it was too expensive—had found a budget deal for a four-day trip to Sammy Hagar Land. Before she bought the tickets in early November, she asked me if it was okay that they left. The deal was only valid during the weekend of my final infusion. I told her, "Of course. You guys should go! I'm going to be okay." And I was genuinely excited for them. Throughout my life, they had *never* taken a getaway vacation. (Well, at least until the year before when they took a similar package trip to Cancun.) I was pleased my mom was finally allowing herself to use her well-earned pay to indulge herself so she and my dad could see places they had never seen. (Throughout my life, she has worked to send much of her earnings to our grandma and family in Peru.)

The blood pressure monitor deflated as Vilma squeaked her stool closer to my arm.

"You know, I read your card," she said, raising her head to look at me. "And it made me teary."

"Awww."

"It's hard—" she said before she looked away, then stared down at the syringe. I murmured. I presumed she was referring to her job in response to what I had written.

Here's what I wrote:

Noreen, Shannon, Vilma, Marva, Consuelo, Dolores, Raquel, Faina, and anyone else at 4C I've forgotten (forgive me, please),

Where to begin, when words like these will always fall short of what I want to express, namely the gratitude, the deep admiration I have for each of you. I am so grateful for the care, for the support and positivity you've given to me and the other patients at 4C. I have always, always known that I can expect this from you; you may shrug it off and think, "That's my job," but in this trying time of my life, it has been beyond comforting to know that I could always count on you.

So this is my teeny-tiny way of saying thank you to each of you. I wish I could give you all a big, big hug. Each of you is sweet and caring in your own ways, and I will always wish you much joy. I'm writing a memoir about this strange period in my life, and I promise you that after I dedicate it to my parents, you all will be the ones I dedicate it to. I'm devoted to writing this book, getting it published someday so I can give you a copy and more thanks. I don't think it's an effect from the chemo (my fix!), but you're angels to me. Thank you, with all my heart.

Very sincerely,

Juan Alvarado Valdivia

(MRN 01721049)*

---

* I included my medical record number because I was afraid the nurses wouldn't

I glanced over at Vilma while she pushed the chemo into me, then turned away. It was always an intensely intimate act to witness—as though man were watching God give him life with a touch from his fingertip. I closed my eyes through the Last One.

Soon after, Connie walked by on her way to attend to one of her patients. She beamed at me, said I was "graduating." I smiled and bowed my head in the oh-shucks way I had done since I was a boy. Though I felt a quiet "woo-hoo!" inside of me, I didn't think it was fitting to celebrate my final infusion in front of the other patients: the middle-aged Russian lady, the vigorous-looking Asian man in his mid-forties, the blue-collar guy who was joking with the nurses for his first infusion, or the old Chinese woman with the gray knit hat whom I had seen wheeled into the ward since I began my infusions. I couldn't celebrate in front of them because I didn't know how long they had to go with their treatment. Or if they would make it through okay. Though I believed I would survive, I could not be certain at that moment, either, so there wasn't much to truly celebrate.

Vilma took off the inflatable cuff, the IV needle from my arm, and bandaged it.

"You're done!" she said.

"Thank you," I said as I bent over to slip my shoes back on. I stood and teetered over to the bathroom a few feet ahead of me. Once inside the airplane-sized bathroom, I slid the folding curtain door behind me. I unzipped my fly. I felt a bad cough coming. My stomach felt sour as it always did right after treatment, but I could feel that it wouldn't be a typical nauseous chemo cough. I bent over the toilet just as I heaved. Some of it splashed on the black slacks I was wearing. It was the only time I vomited right after an infusion. I tried to muffle my post-retch coughs since the other patients or nurses could easily hear through that thin door.

"Are you all right? Did you throw up?" I heard Vilma ask.

"I'm okay," I said, turning the faucet on to splash my face and gargle.

---

remember which former patient had written that card for them (that is, if they kept such tokens, which I'm guessing they did). Once I decided to include the number, I laughed to myself when I thought of it as an homage of sorts to the brilliant 2006 German film *The Lives of Others*. Specifically, I thought of the moment when Dreyman the playwright dedicated his book to the Stasi officer who used to spy on him by using his former officer number in the epigraph.

Fuck. The new guy must have heard. Quite a welcome to Chemo Land. After I cleaned myself up as swiftly as I could, I looked in the mirror. My face was unhealthily pale. Bags under my eyes. I shook my head and made a faint grin, grateful this nasty-ass shit was over when it was beginning to take a toll.

Once I stepped out, I grabbed my shoulder bag. There were no nurses in sight. I opened the door into the infusion room and closed it behind me. (That was the one time the doors into the infusion room were shut.) In the hallway, I found myself hesitant to leave without saying good-bye to someone. Then Vilma stepped out from the nurse's lounge at the end of the hall.

"Big hug?" she asked.

I walked over to her. During my eleventh infusion—which she also administered—I had learned that Vilma had worked at San Francisco General for twenty years. I embraced her tightly, rested my chin on her shoulder. "Thank you," I said, then left before I got teary.

Outside the hospital lobby, the midday sun shone over the Mission. I paused, breathed in the vista, and listened to the humdrum of people filing in and out of the hospital. It felt like listening to the ocean's lapping waves. Paola rolled up in her car. She smiled as I gave her a wave.

"Congratulations," she said as I stepped into the car.

"Thanks, sweetheart."

We leaned over the parking brake to embrace and kiss before we rode off.

Bad Question? (Or Bad Relationship?)

PAOLA AND I stepped into her flat after dinner at Pad Thai Restaurant. We were eager to dash up the stairs to her bedroom. Near the tail end of dinner, our waiter asked if we would be interested in dessert. We gave each other a quizzical look before deciding to pass. Then, with a cocked eyebrow, I told Paola one of my classic postdinner lines. I said, "I'm, uh, *looking forward* to having dessert at your place, if ya know what I mean." Paolita raised a brow and asked, "Oh, really?" Then I followed with something ridiculous: "Are ya lookin' forward to having some . . . Peruvian chorizo?" She rolled her eyes and shook her head in an oh-brother way.

As we ascended the stairs, I was super tempted to give her butt— that sweet bottom I loved with a fervor—a playful smack as I often did. However, Paola and I had mutually agreed, after she broke up with me near the end of September, that I should stop doing that so much. I think we were both afraid that it was symptomatic of some fundamental lack of respect I had for her (though I rather enjoyed it when she smacked my butt, which was rare), but I had told her on a number of occasions that my hands were like magnets drawn to her rump. Every once in a while, I would act out this magnetism, my hands trembling as they drew closer to her tush as if they had a will I could not control. I even misquoted Homer J. Simpson on a number of occasions, telling Paolita that she had "a butt that won't stop." We usually laughed at these antics.

Once in her bedroom, we shut the door behind us. Paola took off her coat and tossed it on her business chair, which was characteristically covered with a pile of discarded clothes. Once I placed my shoulder bag in its usual spot near her bed, I stepped over to Paola. She stood at the foot of her bed. I wrapped my arms around her waist. We kissed as I pulled her tight against me.

"Oooph," I said, "it's getting *awfully* warm down there."

Paola laughed.

"Settle down there, cowboy. You've gotta save that for later!"

"Oh," I said, pulling her hand and pressing it against the bulge in my pants, "there'll be *plenty* for later. Don't you worry. See what you've already done for me?"

She giggled, stepping in to kiss me while she rubbed my cock.

"I'll be back," she said, opening her bedroom door.

"Don't take long!"

I walked over to her nightstand to flick on her Hello Kitty lamp. Then I turned off her overhead light. The room was suffused with soft light. I untied my shoes and took off my socks, placing them neatly beside my bag. I considered taking off my button-down shirt, but I decided to keep it on so that Paola and I could enjoy unbuttoning it. A minute or two passed while I sat expectant on the edge of her bed.

Once I got bored, I began to look around her room. Since it was right in front of me, I skimmed her bookshelf. The self-help books. Books I had lent or given to her. Ones on Latino culture. Books written by her Mills College mentor, Cuban American writer Cristina Garcia. (Paola did not appreciate it when I commented on how hot her teacher was.) Books by Octavio Paz, Junot Díaz, Sandra Cisneros, John Steinbeck, Ernest Hemingway, and Tobias Wolff. I peered at the top shelf where she kept her DVDs and a clutter of knickknacks. The DVD copy of my short film *My Dream of Her* was there, next to her Pilates DVDs. (I know, what a terrible title—sounds like a cheesy soft porn flick.) Two months before, Paola expressed an interest in watching it. I brought the copy and left it on her bed because she didn't express an interest in viewing it with me. I didn't want to be pushy about her watching it. Since then, I noticed it a number of times on the top of her bookshelf. But as I sat there and waited for her, I realized that it was in the same exact space it had always been.

Paola strolled back into the room. She smiled as she walked over to her dresser, giving my thigh a squeeze in passing. I watched her put something away in a drawer.

"Hey, have you seen my movie yet?" I asked, all casual, as if I were asking for the time. She was leaning her head to the side, unfastening an earring. A heavy silence filled the room.

"No."

I took a deep breath and looked away, down at the floor.

"Are you mad at me?" she asked.

"Paola, it took me three years to finish that movie," I said, my voice not so soft and flirty like before. "You're the one who said you wanted to see it, so I left it for you, thinking you would have seen it by now."

"I've been really busy lately, Juan!"

"Busy? Too fucking busy to see a *twelve-minute* movie I made? You mean to tell me in the two months you've had it, you couldn't take twelve minutes of your time to watch it, *especially* after I told you how much it hurt my feelings when you didn't read my submission for our group? I mean, have you learned and tried to change *anything* since we broke up? You talked about doing things to make each other feel special, to make each other know that we really care. And what? You can't even take an interest in my work when you know how much it means to me?"

"It's not like I meant to hurt your feelings."

When she said that, I snickered and rolled my eyes. That was a line that Paola frequently offered whenever she did or didn't do something that subsequently upset me. I always despised that response. It felt like such a cop-out—a way for her to avoid giving an apology and taking any responsibility for the lack of consideration that she had shown. "Sorry" often felt like such a difficult word for her to utter.

"That doesn't matter!" I said. "You're a bright person, and you've been around me long enough to know better. That's bullshit. I have a right to be upset with you right now."

That was Nhat Hanh's teachings on anger coming into play. One of the first things he wrote that resonated with me was that one should not deny one's anger. There's no sense in pretending it isn't there. Bottling up one's anger typically exacerbated that emotion. What was key was *how* you dealt and took care of your anger, your hurt feelings—as though it were a pouting child to be extra gentle with.

I snatched the DVD case and shoved it into my bag.

"You should know better, Paola," I continued, my voice lowering. "You're the one who told me that you wanted to work on showing more affection since you said it's always been a problem for you."

245

"Okay, I'm sorry! Sorry I haven't seen your film. You never told me you wanted it back by some point."

"I didn't. I was just hoping that you would have taken the time to see it by now."

I sat with my back to her, hunched over the edge of her bed. We were quiet for some time. Then she asked what I wanted to do—if I wanted to stay. I told her I would be willing to stay if we were both committed to getting over that not-so-pleasant discussion. Paola didn't want me to leave, and I didn't want to. And so I stayed. I was disappointed, though, sullen that our otherwise delightful evening had taken such an unwanted and unexpected turn. My previously inflamed libido was kaput. I had no desire to be amorous with her, but I stayed because if we wanted to be a couple—and we were struggling to remain one—we *had* to weather such exchanges. We had to get better at that. It was foolish for us to continue to believe that couples that stayed together were ones that rarely argued. Maybe for a few couples this was true, but I was beginning to understand that such couples, in all likelihood, were a rare, rare exception.

I'm not sure what we did afterward. Paola probably slipped into her pajamas while I lay on her bed, reading her latest *New Yorker* issue. After some time had passed, after my disappointment had faded enough, she chitchatted and snuggled up to me until I felt like reciprocating her affection. And then we made love, turned off the lights, and went at it again in the morning before she dressed for work.

When we left to walk to her bus stop (I would always wait with Paola until her bus arrived; for me, it was a beautiful way to begin our mornings), I didn't leave my DVD.

I didn't trust her enough.

In a few weeks, Paola would be leaving town yet again—for three weeks. She was going to visit her family for Christmas, then travel to Portugal and Spain with her roommate, Daisy. They would be there for New Year's and the first weeks of 2010.

It was around that time that I began to question if I was with Paola out of costumbre, out of geographic convenience, or because she sort of stayed with me through a tumultuous time in my life.

But I had no answers.

Here We Go Again

IT STARTED WITH our writers' group meeting held at my home a few days before Christmas. The afternoon sun seeped into the living room where we had gathered. Mimosas were flowing. As was the red wine. After Paola, Lisa, Scott, Amol, and I discussed our group submissions, we guffawed and bullshitted. We were spirited as we began to clean up. I sped over to the kitchen with two empty wine bottles in hand, grinning from my drunkenness.

"All right, so that's it?" Lisa asked.

"Let's go to a bar!" I shouted as I opened the back door to our recycling bins. I didn't think any of them would take up my suggestion that early in the day.

"Where should we go?" Lisa asked.

"Are ya serious?" I asked, back in the living room. "I was just kidding."

"Nah, I'm serious. Where should we go?"

"Let's go to Bliss!" Paola said.

A few hours and several drinks later, Paola, Lisa, Scott, and I were putting our hands together like the Power Rangers. We pledged to finish the first drafts of our respective books by that coming July. It was dark by then. Probably six in the evening. At the bar, I had fueled myself with two or three beers, an appletini, and a shot that Paola had told me—with affection—not to drink, to which I gave a wave of my hand before I downed it.

Then I laid into Paola.

I don't know what prompted my lecture. My self-righteous interrogation. Lisa and Scott were a stool away at the end of the bar, immersed in conversation. Paola sat next to them while I stood beside her, leaning into the bar counter.

"What are you doing with your life, huh?" I slurred, staring into Paola's eyes. Her face was no more than two feet from mine. "You studied journalism and have been writing all these years to, what, work for some business paper? How are you contributing to the good of this world?"

"But I'm—"

"How is the work that you do benefiting this world, Paola? The people who read and subscribe to your paper are a bunch of rich fucking business owners who are just trying to keep up with what's going on so they can stay rich. How does that make a positive difference to our world?"

"But they're the people who are creating jobs—jobs that put food on the table—"

"Pffft. Whatever."

(This is where it gets nauseating for me to remember. I might as well have been hoisted onto a goddamn throne with a big crown on my head.)

"At least *I'm* trying to do something good for this world," I said, tapping a finger to my chest. "I'm writing grants, looking for ones to apply to so that our food pantry can feed poor people in West Oakland, so that kids in that neighborhood can have an arts education. I know it's only part time, and I'm not saying I'm fucking great at what I do, but at least I can go to bed at night with a clear conscience, knowing that at least *I'm trying* to do something good."

Paola started to cry. I remember looking over at Scott and Lisa. I was surprised to see that neither of them came to Paola's defense. Soon after, we left the bar.

We walked a few blocks to a sit-down restaurant. We were in dire need of food. Somewhere during that stroll—as if a mean-spirited devil had leapt off my shoulders, his work done for the night—I realized how hurtful and insensitive I had been with my words. It was as if I had sobered up and realized how critical I was of Paola. My insides constricted.

At the restaurant, when Scott and Lisa's attention drifted, I looked over at Paola with beseeching eyes. "I'm so sorry, Paola, I'm so sorry," I said in a low voice so neither of our friends could overhear. Paola looked back with pained, mournful eyes. I snuck in this apology a few times over dinner. At one point, she rightly called me an asshole. My heart felt like it was being squished.

Once we left the restaurant, Paola dropped us off until I was the only one left. She drove me home. She came inside to pick up her laptop, which she had left thinking we would return from the bar so she could spend the night. She didn't want to say a word to me. From the hallway, I watched her leave, thinking, *My god, this is how it is going to end.* This had happened before. Two years before, drunk on sake, I had chased off my then girlfriend, pissed that she was an hour late for our date due to traffic that was no fault of her own. I watched her walk out of the Japanese restaurant without me, our brief relationship over.

After Paola left, I flopped on my bed. I stared at the ceiling with a feeling of dread twisting my stomach. This was it. I had fucked up. Again. I texted then called Paola, begging to come over to her place so I could apologize further and explain myself. But there were no responses. I curled up on my bed with phone in hand, staring blankly at it, waiting and waiting for a response.

To my relief yet complete fear, Paola eventually returned my call. I begged to see her. She told me she didn't want to talk to me, so we hung up.

And so it was complete: I had destroyed yet another relationship.

And I had allowed my drinking to aid it, yet again.

Early the next morning, I jolted awake from a nightmare in which I was yelling and criticizing Paola—much like I had done the night before. I was a jittery mess. It was too early to call, so I wrote her an e-mail, pleading for her to meet me later. Late in the morning, she called.

"Are you home right now?" she asked.

"Yes," I said, stomach in free fall. "I just—sent you an e-mail."

"I know. I read it. Can I come over? I left my laptop charger in your living room."

When Paola knocked on the door, I gingerly descended the stairwell in my robe. I was afraid I would miss a step and tumble down. My heart felt like it had thumped up to my throat. The sun's light made me squint when I opened the door. She was dressed in a blouse and jeans.

I made a note of this because I feared it might be the last time I would see her. She was scowling at me as she held the books and movies I had lent her.

Grimacing, I held the door open for her. We walked up to my bedroom. I closed the door.

"I'm breaking up with you and giving these back," she said, holding out the books and movies. I shook my head and took them.

"Please don't," I whispered, staring at my bare feet. I could feel my eyes well up.

"Please don't *what*?"

"Please don't leave."

She stood with her hands on her hips while I continued to hang and shake my head, thinking, over and over, *How could I have let this happen?*

"Please don't leave me, Paola," I said, tears falling down my cheeks, my chest heaving as I buried my face in my hands. She put her arms around me.

"I'm so sorry, Paola. I'm so sorry."

She stepped back. I wiped the tears from my eyes, my nose filled with snot. When I looked at her, I could see she was surprised. Her eyes were no longer hard like they were when I opened the door.

"Well—I knew I was still capable of crying," I said. "I knew I still had it in me."

"I have to go," she said.

"I know."

"I'm sure we'll be in touch."

"Yeah," I said, nodding. "I'll walk you to the door."

At the door, we waved and said good-bye. I felt a tremendous sense of relief in knowing that it would not be the last time I would ever speak to her.

After that drinking-episode-gone-wrong, I became afraid to drink around Paola. Afraid of putting myself in an inebriated state where such critical thoughts could come blaring out of my mouth. I was scared of saying something that could harm her. After a fight or an argument, I would sometimes lay awake in bed well into the night with a heart that felt like a smoldering lump of coal. I never felt such anguish for any other girlfriend I ever had. Not even close.

By that point—though I didn't know it then—our relationship was irreparable. A seesaw mess. Once she returned from her trip, Paola and I continued our dysfunctional relationship—on again, off again—for months and months. Throughout that time, our hearts were committed to each other even though she was unable to make a stronger commitment that I felt we needed in hopes of building a new foundation for a healthy relationship.

After our latest makeup, Paola would, on occasion, accuse me of being afraid to be alone. I always told her that wasn't quite the case. When we first dated, I would feel a calm come over me when we were together. A sense of peace filled me when we would hold each other. I just wanted that back. And I sorely wanted to be the good partner I believed I could be.

The Zapper

THE DAY AFTER Paola almost broke up with me again, I had a cancer-filled day scheduled: a morning appointment with Dr. Jaworski at San Francisco General, then an afternoon meeting with Dr. Kirsch at UCSF's Mt. Zion campus. I invited my family to attend the latter appointment, including Carmen, who was in town for the holidays. I was pleased that Carmen would be able to step past the waiting room to see a part of the cancer world that had become my life. I wanted her to be a part of it. I was also pleased that my family would get to meet Dr. Kirsch. I wanted them to be assured that I was in good care.

Dr. Jaworski was sharply dressed when he led me to his small exam room in Ward 86.

"How are you doing?" he asked, perfectly enunciating each word in his Polish accent that endeared me to him. "Have you recovered from all the bad things we've done to you?"

We chortled.

Once we got past our oncologist-patient formalities, Jaworski scooted closer on his rolling chair. He went over the printed results of the pulmonary tests I took on December 8, four days after my last infusion. The lung functions they tested had noticeably declined compared to the exams I had taken before I began chemotherapy. He told me it was to be expected that my lungs would not pack the punch they had before I underwent chemotherapy.

I nodded as Dr. Jaworski explained all this to me. I was pleased at the care he demonstrated in going over those results with me. As a practitioner, he had improved since I came into his care. Since the screw-up over the shortening of my chemotherapy, he had apologized to me. He explained the error he made in arriving to his decision to shorten my treatment: he had failed to look at the results of my first PET scan, which showed my tumor at its largest, at a size that warranted six cycles of ABVD chemotherapy.

Jaworski turned to grab a sheet from the table behind him.

"Now your CT scan . . . came back fine," he said. But the tone in his voice had changed. He sounded grave. "The mass has continued to shrink, but there was one . . . weird thing."

I took a breath and straightened in my chair.

"Since your PET scan on September 22, they found a swollen lymph node off the right side of your trachea. It's probably nothing, but we will obviously have to monitor it."

He handed me copies of both reports. He knew I liked having them, despite the medical jargon that was confounding to decipher.

When he asked if I had any questions, I told him about my right pinky finger. It had swollen around the ring I wore on it. I asked Jaworski why it had swollen, why my fingers had darkened around the knuckles. He was unsure why the chemotherapy had produced those effects, then bent forward to squeeze my calves for "systemic swelling," but he told me I was okay.

Then I asked him the question I was afraid to ask but had to.

"Can that swollen lymph node off my trachea be cancerous?"

"Yes, of course it can," he said. "It's probably from an infection, or from the damage caused to your lungs by the bleomycin. Your respiratory system is a little unstable and weakened right now, especially after six cycles of chemotherapy. I think it's a result of that, especially since your PET scan from a few months ago showed that your mediastinal mass is not active. The damage on your body is cumulative, so it's probably nothing. But we'll keep an eye on it."

I nodded. I was scared. By then, I had been taught to fear *any* unusual bodily occurrence—like the first swollen lymph node, or the subsequent ones. I did my best to focus on the positives in his assessment instead of putting much credence on the worst-case scenario.

Later in the afternoon, I sat in a small waiting room in Mt. Zion's basement. (Charlie Lustman was correct in noting that radiation treatments are always administered in hospital basements—to keep most people from them.) Sporting a floral green gown I felt kind of cutesy in, I took a seat facing the door. Five other people sat and stood in the tight quarters. Like 4C, it looked like I would be the kiddo among the patients. The other men—an Asian guy and two white men—were middle-aged. One guy had shoulder-length peppered hair and a weathered face, like the kind you saw on people who have lived on the streets. Two middle-aged women accompanied him.

Before long, a woman in a white smock opened the door. She called over the long-haired man. Seconds later, the door opened again. A man in his sixties shuffled in. He gave a chuckle, then said, "Heh, back in the waiting room." He gingerly eased himself into the seat that had just been vacated. He had a bruised, ragged-looking gray splotch on his right cheek. It looked like a sickly patch of skin seen on zombies. Marker spots were etched around it like a target sign: [ ]. Inside, I gulped like cartoon characters do when they're nervous.

I grabbed a *New Yorker* from the stand beside me. I took a few calming breaths. I glanced through the table of contents and crossed my leg as though I were on vacation at a hotel bar halfway across the world with a savory tropical cocktail at my side. I flipped to the Shouts and Murmurs column. The goal was to appear as though I were calm, not freaked out by my strange surroundings, but I had to reread the first paragraph several times before I comprehended anything it said.

The door opened. A woman in a white smock called my name. I followed her out into the hall. She introduced herself as Dr. Kirsch's assistant while he stood in the hallway. He wore a button-down shirt and tie in a relaxed manner that made it seem as if that's how he dressed outside of work. He was in his sixties with short, curly black-and-gray hair. His dark eyebrows were bushy in a grandfatherly way.

"Hi, Juan," he said, extending his hand. "It's been a long time since we've met.

"Yes, it's been a long time—since June."

We walked side by side down the hall.

"Do you want your father to join us?" he asked.

"Yeah. Can my mom join us, too? This isn't sexist, is it?"

Dr. Kirsch gave a laugh.

"Yes, of course she can join us."

We waited in the hallway while his assistant fetched my family. Dr. Kirsch introduced himself to them before we crammed into an examination room. I hopped up on the exam table as Dr. Kirsch leaned into the counter behind him. Once we settled into our seats, he asked if I had any questions for him. I didn't, so he turned to my family and asked them. Carmen sat quietly. My parents looked at each other. Mom looked at me before turning to him.

"No, Dr. Kirsch," my mother said. "We don't have any questions for you, thank you."

Kirsch went on to explain the short- and long-term possible effects of radiation treatment. They included: heart disease, lung damage (which could hinder my ability to endure physical activities over a long period of time, such as running a marathon), thyroid problems (since my throat area would be in the radiation field and the radiation mask could not fully shield it), and possible recurrences of cancer.

After the word "cancer" was uttered, I could see this super-worried expression come over my mother's face. Her lips pursed together. Her eyes looked frantic and wounded, like she was on the brink of tears.

"What kind of cancer can he probably get?" she asked.

"Now, I didn't say *probably*," Dr. Kirsch said. "I never said that he will 'probably' get cancer. I did not say that."

He turned to me and asked if I smoked. "No," I said.

Dr. Kirsch turned back to my mom to explain that the kind of cancers I am at risk of developing are organ based, such as lung cancer. But since I don't smoke, he explained that I shouldn't develop that form of cancer. With a calm voice, he continued to tell my parents that the odds of developing cancer from radiation were lower than not getting treatment and relapsing. The pros and cons, in his professional expertise, made it worthwhile to receive radiation treatment.

When I met Dr. Kirsch back in June, he told me the same thing. He had treated cancer patients with radiation for over twenty years at one of the top cancer treatment facilities in the country. After I met him, I could have gone to Stanford to seek a second opinion, but I never doubted him. From the moment I met him, I sensed this uncanny, undeniably soothing spirit emanating from him. Though it was difficult to explain at first (because it was mostly intuitive), I could tell he was a healer. And he was so self-assured, considerate, and in full control of our meetings. Every interaction I had with him afterward only cemented that perception.

I asked if his department would check in with the oncology department at San Francisco General after I completed radiation treatment. Kirsch explained that I would have to see them for "a long time." Once treatment was completed, and my cancer would presumably be in remission, I would have to do follow-up appointments with the oncology department every three months, then every six months, then every year until I was considered to be in complete remission, after five years.

"What about the swollen lymph node by the right side of my trachea?" I asked. "The one that has shown up on my last CT and PET scans. Will the radiation take care of that area as well?"

"Our radiologists don't know what it is," he said. "It doesn't make sense that your cancerous mass is shrinking but that lymph node has grown. Now, remember, that lymph node has never shown up as active."

"PET active?" I asked.

"Yes, PET active [which meant that the lymph node did not light up on the PET scan like cancerous cells would]. If you want, I can show it to you?"

"Yeah, that'd be great."

"That lymph node is close to your mass so I'm going to treat it as well."

I felt a big "phew" when he said that.

"Well—any more questions?" Dr. Kirsch asked us with a faint smile. My mother no longer had that worried expression. We all shook our heads.

"All right, let's get the ball rolling," Dr. Kirsch said, looking at me.

I followed him into his workspace. After he showed me a juxtaposition of the PET scans taken back in June and late September, which clearly showed that the lymph node had grown, a nurse escorted me to a room with a CT scan machine. She ran a quick scan to pinpoint my cancerous mass, then instructed me to continue to lie on the treatment table. One of Dr. Kirsch's assistants was warming up the firm plastic they would use to make my radiation mask. She warned me that it would be a bit hot and tight while it molded around my face. She walked off and brought back a piece of clear plastic that looked like something between an upside-down salad bowl and a speed ramp for toy cars. She had me take off my gown.

"Okay, now we need you to lie back with your neck stretched over this," she said.

I eased back into the plastic piece. My neck fit perfectly into its groove. She asked me to stretch my head back even further until it felt like my neck was being stretched. As I stared at the ceiling from a canted angle, it dawned on me that I was in a prime position to have my throat slashed. Then I heard some approaching footsteps.

"Very good, very good," Dr. Kirsch's voice said. "Your job today is to be a statue."

"Okay," I said.

"Once we make your mask, you'll be done for today. Then we'll have you come in next week so we can do a dry run before we start your treatment."

While I stared at the ceiling, I saw a dark cloth—like a plastic net—swoop down over my face. It was hot like a steaming towel. I heard fastening sounds—snap, snap, snap—around my head. I could barely see through its netting. I was hyperventilating. The firm plastic was fastened so tightly over my face that I could feel my jacked-up heartbeat pulsing from the veins on my neck as it pressed against the mask.

"All right, just hold still," the nurse said.

Get it off, get it off, get it off, get it off, get it off, get it off, get it off, get it off, get it off, get it off!

During the course of my life, I have been in a ridiculously crammed metro train in Santiago, Chile; been squished in my share of buses in Arequipa; and endured hours amid a humid sea of humanity at rock-concert mosh pits, my elbows and forearms jammed into my body. But I never felt like I couldn't handle such tight quarters. Until they molded that radiation mask over my face.

Once I stopped gasping for breath, I began to breathe a little easier through the tiny holes in the plastic mask. At one point, I thought I was going to scream for them to take it off. I was upset the nurse didn't warn me that they were going to Saran-wrap that firm plastic over my face at the moment they did. I doubt it would have made it any easier.

When my family and I exited the hospital, I told Carmen I nearly freaked out when they made my mask. Up until then, I thought radiation treatment would be a cinch compared to the nausea-yucky-nastiness of chemo. How would I make it through one session—let alone twenty—without freaking the fuck out from that radiation mask?

Buzz Buzz

THE FOLLOWING WEEK, I returned to Mt. Zion for my "dry run" of radiation treatment. While sitting in the men's waiting room reading a *New Yorker*, I saw a middle-aged man walk in holding a white plastic mask. It was large enough to cover his face and shoulders. Two pieces of scotch tape formed an "X" on the neck area.

"They're letting me take this home," he said, holding it up as though it were a first-place trophy. The four of us sitting in the waiting room chuckled as he walked into the locker room.

"Honey, look what I got!" said the adorable old man who sat beside me, pretending to be the man with the mask. I laughed. He had short white hair, bushy eyebrows, and glasses that Buddy Holly would have found befitting. In a few days, I would befriend him.

The waiting-room door swung open. A middle-aged woman with stylishly cropped blonde hair held it. She called my name.

"Hi Juan, I'm Pat," she said, extending her hand as I walked into the hallway with her. "I will be your patient advocate." Pat was my height and appeared to be in her mid-fifties. Her breath had a potent whiff of coffee to it.

We walked into a dimly lit hallway. We stopped outside a tiny passage replete with computers and monitors. At a glance, it looked like a tiny broadcast television room. A petite, cute Asian woman with her hair tied in a ponytail stood there.

"Juan, this is Maria. She will be your radiation therapist," Pat said.

"Hi Juan. It's nice to meet you!" Maria said, stepping forward to shake my hand.

After Maria verified my identity and took my weight on a scale beside two blue doors with a large yellow-and-black radiation sign that read "DO NOT ENTER. RADIATION FIELD," Pat escorted us into the room that read "Oncor 4."

The room had a cavernous quality to it. A dark wooden floor. Dim fluorescent lighting that one would expect to see at a morgue. The dominant presence in the room was a large white machine that stood against the back wall. It looked like an upside-down "L," or an old phone fit for a giant. Beside it dangled a remote control of sorts, attached to a Twisstop cord. Ah, this must be the machine that's gonna fry me, I thought. Beneath the protruding part of the machine, in the middle of the room, was a table that rested over what looked like the expanding bellows of an accordion.

"All right, let's have you sit up here," Pat said, patting the clothed table.

I hopped up on it while Maria scurried over to a corner. She brought back a red foam cushion to place beneath my legs. Pat helped to lay me back so my neck was bent over the piece of plastic used to hold my head straight while my radiation mask was molded. She put a blanket over my torso, then strapped me to the table with my arms tucked against my sides. While she did this, Pat explained that this was the routine they would follow every morning for my treatments.

"Okay, you ready? We're going to put on your mask," Maria said.

"Okay."

Standing at my sides, Pat and Maria brought the white plastic mask down over my face. Like when the mold of my face was made, I heard snapping sounds all around my head. With each snap, the mask tightened. I could barely see or breathe through it. My heartbeat spiked. I could feel the veins in my neck pulsing against the mask. Then, like a slow zoom-in, they raised the table I rested on toward the machine I lay beneath. Soon after, they lowered me back down to snap off the mask.

"You'll be in and out of here in fifteen minutes or less," Maria said as I sat up.

"Wow, really? Is *this* where I'm getting zapped?" I thought the radiation treatment machine would resemble a cathode ray gun, or a sci-fi death ray.

"Yup! You'll probably only be in here for a few minutes."

I'll be damned, I thought.

"Ya know, when I told my friends I'd be getting radiation, I tried to make it fun by giving it a name like the Zapper. But I'm still not sure if that's the best name."

Maria crinkled her eyebrows and looked off pensively.

"Hmmm, I'd say it's more like 'buzz buzz.'"

I giggled.

Pat escorted me back to the men's dressing room to wait for Dr. Kirsch. Maria and Pat struck me as excessively cheerful spirits, but I was happy to be around their sunny presence. From a logistics standpoint, however, I was still a little freaked out about this whole getting-zapped-with-cell-destroying-subatomic-particles business. To make matters worse, while I was locked into the mask and raised toward the ceiling, I had two thoughts that were discomforting in tandem:

1. I will be receiving my treatment in the hospital's basement beneath five floors of steel and concrete.
2. THIS IS EARTHQUAKE COUNTRY!

When I sat with Dr. Kirsch in his exam room, I told him I nearly had a panic attack when the radiation mask was clamped over me, my arms pinned against my sides.

"We're not here to torture you," he said. "We're putting on that mask and tying your arms so that I know we're hitting the right spot."

But I already knew that. None of them struck me as the sadistic type. Quite the opposite.

"You won't feel a thing from the radiation," he said. "As we continue with treatment, you might feel some fatigue. And your chest—the area where we'll be treating you—might get a little pink and irritated, like a sunburn."

I nodded.

"Any more questions?" he asked.

"Ummm, it's a . . . silly question," I said, shaking my head.

"Nah, c'mon. There are no silly questions here," Kirsch said with a wry grin.

I told him I was a little concerned that my radiation treatments would be administered in the hospital's basement. It had occurred to me that I would be in a pretty shitty spot if an earthquake happened, tied down and locked to that machine. I told him I had even briefly fantasized about bringing "a pocket chainsaw or something" in case I needed to cut myself out of that mask.

"I know that's absurd—and I know I'm a little crazy," I said, putting up my hands. "But I'm a little concerned."

Dr. Kirsch looked bemused.

"If there was an earthquake, Pat and Maria would run in and release you," he said.

"Oh that's good. There's a protocol!"

He looked like a teacher trying not to laugh in front of the class after a student said something ludicrous.

Before I left, I shook his hand with both of mine cupped over his. It was the extra-special handshake I busted out to convey extra-special gratitude. (I believe I picked it up from a priest, years ago, when I was a videographer.) He held the door open and patted me on the back.

"We'll see you next week."

2010: A Strange Odyssey

WEARING BLUE SWEAT pants, a gray hoodie, and my bicycle helmet, I walked down the dark stairwell of my flat hoisting Blue above my shoulder. It was 7 a.m., Monday, January 4, 2010. First day of radiation treatment. My appointments for the rest of that week were at 7:30 a.m. It was the only time slot Pat and Maria could squeeze me into. They had shown me their morning-to-afternoon schedule; it was all booked. Henry Ford would have been proud at the number of people they were bringing in and out to get zapped.

I rolled down 22nd Street to hang a left on Valencia. The streets were empty other than a few joggers and people walking about. It was a smidge chilly. I considered turning back home for a thicker sweater, but I had been everywhere with that hoodie, which my first significant girlfriend had given to me nine years before. I had backpacked through Western Europe, South America, Cuba, the Yucatan, Thailand, and Cambodia with it. Together, we would endure radiation treatment, too.

As I took the elevator to the hospital basement, wiping sweat from my face, I felt proud of myself. My dad had offered to lend me his Toyota Rav4 so I could drive myself to the hospital throughout treatment. Mariana and her husband had offered to take me to and from the hospital. I thanked them but declined their offers. In a suburb like Fremont, my dad needed a vehicle to get around. And I didn't want to hassle Mariana that early in the morning. It was tempting to borrow my dad's SUV, but I wanted to push myself. Man up. In my heart, I believed that the three-mile rides to and from the hospital would nourish me. Strengthen my resolve. Build my resilience. After reading Norman Cousins's *Anatomy of an Illness* the year before, I knew how vital the mind and one's convictions were in the healing process. As long as the treatment did not fatigue me, I was determined to cycle to my appointments. The hard part would be waking up on time since I was a night owl.

The moment I opened the door into the men's locker room, I saw the old man with bushy white eyebrows and Buddy Holly glasses I had seen the week before. He sat on the cupboard bench where the gowns were kept.

"Good morning," he said.

"Good morning to you, too," I said, opening a locker to put my backpack in.

"They're going to have me on chemo for an entire week. Did you have chemo?"

"Yeah, I finished."

"How much did they give you?"

"Six cycles," I said, keeping our conversation to cancer-world jargon.

"What kind of cancer do you have?"

"Hodgkin's lymphoma."

He didn't nod or have a knowing look in his eyes.

"It's a rare one. A blood cancer," I said.

He asked if it was similar to leukemia. I told him I wasn't sure. Then he stood and walked over to me.

"Well, take care of yourself," he said, opening his arms.

"You too," I said, hugging him back. My neck and upper back were damp with sweat, which is why I almost apologized to him when he put a hand on my neck. Once we let go, he opened the door to let himself out. We were smiling, grateful for this unanticipated early morning affection from a fellow cancer fighter.

"I'll see you around," he said, as if we were boarding an all-expenses-paid flight to Maui.

"Take care, man."

In the dimly lit radiation room, I hopped up on the treatment table. Pat and Maria snapped the mask down to the table. It was clamped down over my face so that my eyelashes bent against the mask whenever I blinked. They confirmed that the X-marks on the part of the mask that covered my shoulders were aligned with the green lasers that shot from both sides of the room like laser pointers. After tying me down with my arms pinned to the sides, Maria gave me a horn to hold in my right hand. It was like a clown horn.

"Use it in case you need anything," Maria said.

"Okay," I murmured, barely able to open my mouth.

After they raised me toward the ceiling, beneath that curious-looking part of the machine that hung over the treatment table, Pat and Maria turned to leave.

"We'll be next door in case you need anything, okay," Pat said. "You're doing great."

The lights went off. I heard the door shut.

Once the room became completely dark, I could see a soft white light emitting from the machine hanging over me. It was about two feet away. The light came through a rectangular piece of glass with markings on it that looked like quadrants for measurement. It made me think of a periscope. Since the machine didn't look like a pointy laser out of a sci-fi movie or a James Bond flick, it was difficult to imagine that contraption as the one that would zap my chest. But once I saw that light penetrating through the periscope-like opening, once I saw that square opening of light narrow, then widen, it was clear that that was where I would get a stream of subatomic particles shot at me.

The machine slowly rotated to my left. I was befuddled and mesmerized. It reminded me of the languid, poetic movements of the spaceships in Kubrick's *2001: A Space Odyssey*. That's probably why I began to hear Strauss's "The Blue Danube" play in my head.

Once it rotated out of my peripheral vision, I heard the machine make a buzzing sound as though there was a loud hair clipper behind me. The buzzing lasted for a few seconds. *Oh, I must have just been zapped!*

Then I heard the humming sound of the machine as it gently rotated back in front of me. All the while, the lilting Strauss score in my head became louder while I observed this strange beauty. I was trying to distract myself from the weirdness of it all.

When the machine stopped and produced that *buzzzzzzzzzzzzz* sound again, I focused on the chest area by my tumor. I swore I could feel something—a sliver of heat—as though a magnified beam of sunlight had shot through the room to shine on it. I am not sure if that sensation was simply in my head, but while I got zapped, I imagined a searing laser beam sawing through the cavernous tumor that Mr. Hodgkins and his minions made as their lair. I imagined boulders breaking off, crashing down as they scattered in disarray.

Weeks later, Maria would explain to me that the machine had zapped me with radioactive particles from the back and the front. If it were done twice from a single position, it would have done more damage to my internals.

The buzzing stopped. The door opened. The fluorescent lights flicked on as Pat and Maria walked over to my side. Maria began to unfasten the mask.

"Okay, you're done," she said. "Let me lower you down."

"I'm *done*?"

"That's it."

Once I was lowered, I swung my legs over to hop down on the floor. Maria placed my mask on top of a steel shelving unit against the side of the room. I had never really noticed it before. There were three levels of shelves about ten feet in length. The top shelf was crammed with masks—about ten to fifteen of them. They all had large X-marks taped onto numerous spots: the neck, cheek, skull. Like my mask, each had a long piece of masking tape placed over the upper torso. It had the owner's name and identifying medical-record number written on it. The middle shelf held other wire-mesh masks. Those were shaped to cover other parts of the human body, such as the chest, lower back, or upper thighs.

All those names taking up those other schedule slots suddenly felt more real.

It was sobering to see all those masks.

After Pat escorted me back to the dressing-room area, I went to the bathroom to pee. When I stepped to the sink to wash my hands, I discovered a curious sight reflected back at me in the mirror. My face—forehead, nose, and cheeks—looked like they were covered in fish scales. The mask had made creases all over my face.

"Man," I said to myself. I was perversely tickled that I had physical evidence of just how tight that mask was clamped on me. I took out my cell phone and snapped a pic of my scaly looking face.

The sky was a swirl of lavender when I cycled home along Post Street. The sun was lifting above the skyscrapers in the distance. I marveled at this early morning beauteousness I rarely saw, this unexpected gift I had been graced with.

One down, nineteen to go! I thought when I rolled up to my home. *Six miles down, 114 to go.*

Morning Hugs

THE NEXT MORNING, I opened the door to the men's locker room and saw the same man I had hugged on Monday.

"Hi, how are you?" I asked.

"I'm good, how are you?" he asked.

"I'm good," I said, opening a locker to stuff my backpack in. "What time are you getting here in the mornings?"

"My appointment's at 7:15."

"Ah! No wonder we keep seeing each other."

"So how much do you have to do, guy?"

"Four weeks. And how about you?" I asked, lifting my shirt out to dry the sweat from my chest with a hand towel.

"Seven weeks," he said with a grimace.

"Hmm. And yesterday you said you have to do a week of chemo?"

"Yeah, a week here, then an entire week of chemo. And then . . . about five weeks of radiation."

We were quiet, thinking of something to say. Wasn't exactly conversational material that we longed to delve into. Not an "And how are your grandkids?" sort of conversation.

"Did you just come in from the gym?" he asked. He must have thought this since I was wearing sporty sweat pants and running shoes and was drying sweat on my head. My hair was cropped. In December, I had tried to grow it out once chemo was done, but once it got a smidge long—about an inch or so—it kept falling off in clumps whenever I shampooed. A few weeks later, Jaworski would tell me that it would take *months* for the chemotherapy to cycle out of my body.

"No," I said, grinning. "I just bicycled from home, three miles away."

"Oh wow, so you've been able to handle it well with your chemo treatment?"

"Yeah. Oddly enough, I gained weight during chemo, so it seems like my body handled it pretty well, fortunately."

Then he asked how old I was. When I told him I was thirty, he told me he was seventy. "You're just a baby, a poulette," he said, which made me laugh. He thanked me when I told him he looked good for his age.

He stood from the bench and walked over to me, his arms spread for what quickly became our morning hug routine.

"We're going to make it," he said with a brave grin when we took a step back, our arms still around each other.

I hesitated to respond. His statement, his wish, caught me by surprise. Surviving cancer seemed like a formality for me. Since I was receiving treatment, I would have to be an exception if lymphoma killed me. (At least initially. Surviving five years after diagnosis is a different matter altogether, though I did not know it then.) I was taken aback to be reminded that this was not the case for everyone fighting to be cancer-free.

"We are," I said as we ended our embrace.

"I'll see you later," he said, stepping around me to walk out of the room.

"Take care." I thought it was neat that we had parted from one another without asking each other's name. I was tempted to ask him his name, though.

I walked over to the bench where he had been sitting. The door opened. He peered in.

"Hey, what's your name?"

I smiled.

"Juan."

"I'm David," he said. I stood and walked over to shake his hand with both of mine.

"A pleasure," I said before he left.

When I strolled out of the hospital to unlock Blue (two down, eighteen to go!), I looked at the time on my iPod. It took fifteen minutes on the dot to walk in and out of the hospital for treatment. My second session went down like the previous one, except Maria and Pat must have graduated me to big-boy status since they had not given me an emergency horn to hold. Before they clamped the mask on me, I took a deep breath. It helped to calm me from its claustrophobic tightness.

I felt tired, having slept little more than five hours for the second night in a row. But I was already looking forward to seeing David the following morning.

David was not in the men's locker room the next day. After my treatment, Pat and Maria asked if I wanted to change my appointment time to 8:20 a.m. Before my subatomic-zapping-particle sessions began, I had asked for a later morning time for my treatments. I could start my new appointment time the next day, but I declined. I told them about David and our morning hugs and how I looked forward to them.

Two days later, Friday morning, I awoke in a sweat. My first alarm had not roused me out of bed. I was running late if I wanted to catch David! Instead of taking my usual route down Valencia to avoid climbing the steep hill on Dolores Street, I swiftly pedaled halfway up that hill, then stomped up the rest of the way. By the time I got to the top, which provided a splendid view of the city to the east, I was panting. Once a few cars passed by on the narrow two-lane street, I raced down Dolores Street, through the morning gray. I had to ride the brakes to slow to a twenty-five-mile-per-hour speed, which would give me a marginal shot at evading a car looking to merge onto Dolores from a side street without seeing me, or weave away from a driver's-side door opening in front of me. It was like a gauntlet. Riding it made my heart throb with fear and excitement. Once I made it down the hill, I pedaled as hard as I could to the hospital, running stop signs, even a red light at Market Street once it was safe to cross. The time was 7:22 when I arrived at Mt. Zion.

Drenched in sweat, I whisked into the men's dressing room. As always, David and I bumped into each other in the locker room. He told me he had begun his chemotherapy infusions, which is why he didn't "feel so hot." Pat had told him that the following week I would be coming in at a later time. This pleased me to hear. I presumed she told him I had kept the 7:30 slot that first week so I could see him in the morning.

David suggested that we stay in touch. I was delighted he brought it up first. I handed him my card, which had some outdated info.

"I'm no longer a filmmaker," I said as David sat on the bench and studied it. "And I was never much of a photographer."

"But you're still a writer?" he asked.

"Yeah. Heh, it took me years to figure out that I was one all along."

I told David I was getting my MFA. He told me he was a bit of a bibliophile. He had tremendous respect for writers and would love to read my work. After he asked me who my favorite authors were—a question I have always fumbled (I tend to think in terms of favorite books, though I did blurt out Sherman Alexie, J. D. Salinger, David Foster Wallace, and Tom Robbins)—I asked David where he lived. We were excited to find that we were neighbors: he lived a few blocks away on the other end of Dolores Park. I told him I would be glad to help him with any errands he needed help with. He told me he appreciated it, though he had a partner who was being so supportive of him.

Before I left for my treatment, David graced me with the one thing I wanted that morning: a hug from him—his warmth in my arms.

A Moonlight Serenade

CUE THE SOUND. Track the film camera back, a bit faster than my pace. There I am, in focus, in the middle of the wide-angle frame, wearing a black pea coat, gray slacks, and the loafers I wore to work. It's five o'clock, Thursday evening. Downtown San Francisco, corner of Market and Montgomery Streets. Watch as I part through the crowd funneling past me into the underground tunnels. Now see them through my point of view: a mass of silhouetted figures bathed in golden light, the sun setting behind them past the hills. *This is my life*, I think to myself while I listen to the timeless, lilting melody from Glenn Miller and his big band orchestra through my headphones. *This is the world I'm still a part of.* Now switch to a close-up of my clean-shaven face as the camera continues to track backward. My hair, in its rebirth, is growing again. A contented grin comes over me. *If it weren't for my treatment, I might not have seen this.*

On most occasions, I would have probably felt annoyed to walk against wave upon wave of humanity, hurrying to pile into crowded trains from their tiny cubicles. But I feel graced to be among them as they brush past me. Chirping into their phones. Texting while walking. Marching with expressionless faces. Muffling the world around them with music playing from their headphones.

In my world, in my head, curious thoughts begin to dawn as the sunlight fades on another day. I think to myself, *Someday I want to play and pass this song along to my children, to fill our home with its peaceful rhythm.* I think to myself, *I want to play this song when I leave this town. I want this song to play at my wedding reception. And someday, when my sun is setting, I want to sit and close my eyes and listen to this song fill my heart like the sound of the ocean's waves.*

As I walk down the sidewalk to meet a friend, I play the song again and again—stirring those images, those emotions. This is new for me—the desire to imagine a future.

I play the song again and again and again.

Pedaling with the Wolves

HALFWAY THROUGH MY four weeks of radiation treatment, the weather in San Francisco took a soggy turn. Weather forecasters predicted heavy rain through the middle of January. My parents were concerned about my cycling through the rain. My pop offered me his vehicle again. This time, I accepted.

I figured it would be smart to borrow his Rav4 in case the rain was too daunting. While I wanted to physically push myself during radiation treatment—the stretch run—I also recognized that it might be wise to ease off the accelerator. During this strange period of my life, I had to conserve my energy for healing from the months of treatment (though that understanding did not deter me from drinking like it should have). Besides, I knew I *could* bicycle in heavy rain to the hospital if I had to. On that matter, I had nothing to prove to myself.

With ten treatments down and ten to go, I felt great. To my jolly surprise, I didn't feel the least bit fatigued like I figured I would. (Marva, one of the 4C nurses, once told me, "It took me a while to understand, but chemo makes you sick. Radiation makes you tired.") At times, my throat felt like it had constricted, which made it painful to eat, or even to swallow my own saliva. A few itchy bumps, like hives, had sprouted along my right forearm. Kirsch did not think it was an effect from treatment since that arm was well outside the "plain of radiation." But I figured it was. My final seven infusions were injected into that arm. The veins still looked nasty-purplish.

When Monday, January 18, rolled around, I startled from my alarm. Once I shut it off, I heard the pitter-patter of rain on my window. I rolled up my bamboo blinds. It was pouring outside.

Driving my dad's Toyota Rav4 through the rain felt luxurious. It was warm, effortless to propel forward—a dry experience compared to riding my Bianchi. I was grateful for my dad's generosity. And thankfully I took his offer, because I saw a few street corners that were mini-lagoons. On the drive to the hospital, I saw a handful of bicyclists pedaling through the torrent. Wolves, I called them. I had mad respect for each cyclist that braved the rain and slippery streets.

The next two days were not as rainy. On Wednesday, it sprinkled on the way to the hospital. It made me feel yucky to use that vehicle and expend fuel when I didn't need to. Whenever I saw a cyclist pedaling down the street in their rain gear, I felt like a wimp. *I should be rolling with the wolves!*

So Thursday morning, come drenching rain or sunshiny skies, I was determined to cycle to the hospital. I *knew* I was physically fit to cycle six miles to and from the hospital, rain or shine.* I didn't want to be a wuss about it just because I was at the tail end of cancer treatment.

Donning my rain gear, I pedaled to Mt. Zion. On the ride there, I headbanged a bit while listening to Guns N' Roses and Mötley Crüe. I could proudly give a nod whenever I passed a fellow wolf on two wheels. To my chagrin, the ride was too easy, though I was pleased when it began to drizzle during the final mile. The mist was invigorating as it fell on my face while I pedaled past Alamo Square. The rain felt cleansing.

When Pat looked at my wet hair and asked if I had been caught in the rain, I told her I cycled to the hospital. She gasped.

And as I had anticipated, the warm shower when I returned home was glorious.

It was around this time that I considered seeking depth psychotherapy. My roommate Kelly—who had recently entered therapy—thought I could benefit from it due to my self-reflective disposition and relatively open nature. He painted a therapist as a life coach of sorts, a copilot to

---

* Three years before, during the rainiest March in San Francisco's modern history, I cycled every weekday to and from work. It rained *twenty-five days* that month, but it did not deter me from cycling seven miles each day for my commute. I'm still rather proud of that feat. I always reasoned that such an act built inner resilience.

take along into the depths of one's mind, into the individual worlds we saw, felt, and created. And that sounded great. I was much too biased to look at myself in any form bordering on objective.

Like the stubborn-minded man I can be, I still believed that my rocky relationship with Paola could be saved. The urgency that drove me to seek therapy *was* our relationship. I expected my therapist to tell me what to do about our relationship, to point out where I had failed (though, I had a *fair* idea where I had), to help me nourish and save it.

If that is what I truly wanted, deep down inside.

Farewells

FOR OUR LAST meeting, Dr. Kirsch walked into the exam room wearing a tan-colored tie that dreadfully accompanied his khakis and striped button-down shirt. I figured it was his oh-fuck-it, this-outfit-doesn't-go-together-but-it-makes-me-look-like-a-doctor outfit. Once he sat down, he told me that we were "coming down to the end"—seventeen treatments down, three more to go. After he asked if the Mylanta he had recommended to alleviate the tightness in my throat had worked, he asked if I had any questions. Leaning forward, elbows on my knees, I asked if he had "targeted" the baffling lymph node growing off of my trachea. He assured me he had. I asked if he thought the PET scan scheduled for February 25 was too early to conclusively tell if my cancer had been eradicated. He shook his head, told me he didn't think so.

"After today, I hope I won't be seeing you again," Dr. Kirsch said. "From here on, you'll be following up with San Francisco General."

I nodded.

"What I mean is," he said with a faint grin, "I hope I won't see you *here* again."

"I'm glad you put it that way. I'm glad you didn't mean, 'I hope I'll *never* see you again!'"

He grinned.

"You've done six cycles of chemotherapy. You're going to complete twenty sessions of radiation. We've given you the correct treatment. The odds are good that you will be free of your disease."

I smiled as he stood to shake my hand.

"It was good to see you," I said. He held the door open for me. When I walked into the hallway, I turned back and thoughtlessly said, like the Californian I am, "See ya later." I immediately regretted it. *Wait, I DON'T want to see you later—and certainly not here!*

With the end of treatment within grasp, I began to plot how to celebrate this momentous occasion. Earlier in the month, I had written on my Facebook profile that I was "shopping for a coffin for Mr. Hodgkins." A few of my friends thought it was a good idea to procure a miniature coffin, and they suggested I bury it somewhere. I thought that was too hokey, though. On that same Facebook thread, I mentioned making a Mr. Hodgkins piñata to destroy. My peeps dug that idea. I even searched for a place that made custom piñatas to no avail. Then I imagined it would be cooler to plant a Mr. Hodgkins headstone (Here Lies Fuckface) somewhere so that my friends and family and I could have a dance party over it. The B-52s "Rock Lobster" would be the first jam to get that delicious wackiness going, followed by some potent eighties jams. But then January's heavy rainfall inspired yet another daydream. Though I knew it wouldn't happen, I daydreamt of having a rooftop dance party in the rain to celebrate.

This was all fine and dandy to conjure, but I was still unsure *what* to do in real life.

The following Monday, I celebrated my final day of treatment by asking Pat to snap pictures of me while I was locked into the treatment table. They had switched me to another room with a circular ceiling lit with soft blue lighting, dotted with tiny bulbs to resemble twinkling stars. It looked like the ceiling at a planetarium. I also took my radiation mask home. I considered it a trophy, figured it would make a curious-looking artifact in my room, a token of this period in my life I could and would not forget. Paola and a few of our friends trekked across the bay for celebratory ice-cream sundaes at Fentons Creamery.

And so began Life after Lymphoma-Vanquishing Treatment. The following week, my final semester at Saint Mary's would begin as would my first foray into therapy.

The Big Aside

How can you live a special life without constantly interrogating it?

—SHERMAN ALEXIE, *Ten Little Indians*, 2004

I SAT AND faced Akhila, the attractive woman about my age with curly brown hair whom I had chosen to be my therapist. She sat straight in a dark leather armchair, staring intently at me. A notepad and pen rested on her lap. The room was awkwardly quiet. The only noises I heard were the soft whooshes from passing cars outside the window that allowed light into the study.

"So to start off, why don't you tell me why you're seeking therapy— and what you hope to get from it."

"Well, first of all, I feel like it's a *slight* achievement to be here," I said. My hands were cupped in my lap. "I've never been in therapy. Up until a few months ago, I never even considered it. As far as I can remember, my parents never raised me and my sisters to believe that anyone who went into therapy was *really* fucked up, but that's what I used to think for the longest time."

I went on to tell Akhila that I had come to understand that we are all fucked up to various degrees. (Having desires and living around people will do that to you.) Subsequently, there was no shame in seeking therapy. When I said this, she nodded in an affirming way.

Then I told Akhila that in my thirty years of living on Planet Earth, I must have developed some beliefs and habits that were not healthy. Maybe even detrimental to my well-being. In seeking her help, I hoped to have her guidance in interrogating my thoughts, my feelings, my way of seeing our world.

After I told Paola I was going into therapy, she advised me to come up with three goals. Since Akhila wasn't saying much, just sitting there and staring at me with a pleasant grin that made me uncomfortable (I bet she was terrific at staring contests), I told her I had goals for therapy:

1. To focus on my anger—to figure out why I had self-destructive tendencies, especially around alcohol;
2. To discuss my romantic relationships, since none of them tended to last long;
3. To scrutinize my world view, because I was concerned I had developed some beliefs that were harmful to my well-being.

"Oh and, uh, I also just finished battling cancer," I said. "I was diagnosed last year and finished chemotherapy and radiation treatment last week."

Once Akhila and I notched a few weeks of therapy together, we would come to refer to that glancing mention of cancer as "the big aside." She would even joke about it.

Kelly had recommended the center where Akhila practiced. Their clinicians brought a multifaceted approach to depth psychotherapy, including an emphasis on the spiritual and creative aspects of the self. Akhila's clinical profile on their website stressed her experience with LGBTIQ individuals. She also had vast experience in studying world religions and ecopsychology, which I had never heard of before. I deduced that Akhila's work with the LGBTIQ community, coupled with her mysterious ethnic background, would give her an unspoken but crucial understanding of what it's like to be part of "the others" in society—like a progressive Peruvian American atheist like myself. And lastly, but just as importantly, she was a woman. Given my personal history, being raised by women[*] and having more lady friends than wangs, I figured it would be easier to express my feelings to her instead of a man.

---

[*] On dates, interviews, and during conversations with folks I'm meeting for the first time, I have often jokingly but truthfully told them I was "raised by women." I usually share this tidbit to explain my effeminate nature, why I'm so goddamn sensitive compared to most men, or to joke about why I should be considered prime dating material. But the fact is, I *was* raised in a household with two sisters and no brothers. Throughout my upbringing, I was much closer to my mom than my dad because she was more involved in our lives. At the very least, sharing a bathroom with my two sisters trained me into being a good boy about putting the toilet seat down when frequenting a household with female inhabitants.

At the end of our meeting, Akhila asked if I still wanted her as my therapist. "Yeah," I said, with the assurance of a "hell yeah." I left the office feeling light and excited, knowing we would meet next week for the beginning of our journey through my crazy-ass mind. I was also happy that I could finally make good use of what I had called "the cancer slush fund," the $1,500 in donations my mother's coworkers at Cabrillo Elementary had given her after I was diagnosed to help with my cancer treatment.[*]

On the bike ride home, I felt radiant—as though I was humming with light. Without a doubt, I knew seeking help was a benevolent and necessary act for me. *This* is what I expected from my postlymphoma self.

But I was also happy because my classes started the next day.

---

[*] At first, I did not want to accept their money. When I was first diagnosed, it looked like the Healthy San Francisco program would cover the costs of my treatment. In the prior two years, my mom—who served as a bilingual liaison for the Spanish-speaking parents of the school—had to wait through the summer to see if she still had a job. Thanks to budget cuts in public education (while our country's military expenditures totaled almost half of our nation's federal budget), folks were being laid off at Cabrillo Elementary. There were rumblings that their salaries would have to be renegotiated in the coming school year. My mom's colleagues were not people with ample wherewithal.

But I accepted their gift because my mom implored me to; their generosity was a remarkable act of goodwill my family could not deny. The money was handed to us in a large manila envelope stuffed with checks, money orders, dollar bills, and a large Hallmark card her colleagues signed, sending their love and prayers. My mom and I have their card tucked away.

ON THE FIRST day of the spring semester, I rode Blue to school. The sun glistened on my arms, the wind at my back. While I cycled along the golf course in Moraga, staring out toward the surrounding verdant hillside, it dawned on me that it might be the first ride I ever took to school without a cancerous cell in my body.

During an evening break for our Craft of Fiction class, I shot the shit with a few Nonfictionistas. My classmate Christine asked if I had ridden my bike to school. I was all too eager to tell her I had.

"I think today's ride was the first one I've ever taken to school without cancer!"

"That's amazing!" she said. Though I've had difficulty accepting compliments throughout my life, I embraced that one.

After class, under the starry blanket of night, I cruised down the trail that wove through Lafayette. The town was quiet. All I could hear was the soft whirring sound of the wheels rolling over the pavement. I pitched my head back to stare at the stars. I breathed in the crisp air. Once I passed an orange streetlight, I turned to watch the shadowy outline of the trees along the path as I glided past them. In less than four months my graduate studies would be over. My life—with good health permitting—was in for significant change. So long, student life. So long to my classmates and professors. So long part-time work—and hello student-loan payments. I felt nervous and sad and grateful and eager to carve an altered life in the work world, one surrounded with writing. But those nighttime rides along the Lamorinda hillside, alone with those trees, those stars above me—I knew I would miss them dearly.

HUMP DAY IN the middle of February provided a helluva jolt: Amber called a house meeting to tell Kelly, Crystal, and me that she was moving out. The problem was that she was the master tenant, the only person on our lease. A week later, after an exhausting, contentious, and completely unexpected dispute with Amber over our security deposits (one of her prior roommates had screwed her out of half of the deposit years before, and she hoped we would help her cover part of it), we were told that we all had to vacate Casa 909 by the end of April. The landlords were giving us the boot. With my final semester of grad school already underway, now I had to scramble to move and find a new home.

A few days later, itchy, painful, pus-filled rashes with blisters popped up along my right forearm. A few broke out in clumps by my elbow and armpit. I thought they were hives. This had never happened before. Though they kept refilling with pus, I couldn't stop myself from popping them again and again and again. I came to enjoy the burning sensation it produced.

Despite the pleasant late February weather, I wore a sweater throughout the following days. The red bumps were icky to look at. They looked contagious. I didn't want my classmates or coworkers to stare at them and ask, "What is *that*?" One person I felt comfortable showing them to was David, my buddy from radiation treatment. Since we said good-bye in the men's locker room, we had exchanged a few affectionate, supportive e-mails, then went out for breakfast near the end of February. Though he was no doctor, he thought the rashes were hives, too.

That made complete sense. Never in my life had I felt such anxiety: having to move out during my already hectic final semester of grad school. The nervousness I felt about graduating at the end of May. My topsy-turvy relationship woes with Paola. (I had broken up with her less than a week after Valentine's Day.) The tension I felt at home. But above all, I was worried about my health. I had a crucial PET scan in a few days. On March 2, I would meet with my new oncologist to go over the results. To see if I was lymphoma-free.

There was so much uncertainty in my life.

And there was so little I had control over.

The Best News Ever

RAINDROPS FELL OVER me as I cycled to Ward 86 for my 8:30 a.m. oncology appointment. The sky was a dark, pregnant gray. It had begun to rain the night before. I stayed up well past midnight revising one of the opening chapters for my thesis. Once I lay down in bed, a gentle pitter-patter of raindrops tapped my window. Surprisingly, I fell asleep with ease. By then I had managed to find peace in knowing that I received the treatment my cancerous mass merited. Aside from all the drinking I shouldn't have done, I did what I could throughout treatment. The past could not be reversed. Plus, I took the rain as a sign that tomorrow would bring good news. Absolve me. Grace me with a fresh beginning.

I sat in the crowded waiting room with other Ward 86 patients. Highlighter in hand, I read an essay for one of my classes. My parents were nowhere around. I didn't invite them to accompany me for that all-important meeting. I figured I could handle it on my own, no matter what the results of the PET scan were. Plus, I had a somewhat busy Tuesday ahead of me at school, so I figured I wouldn't have had much time to be with them after the meeting. But not inviting them to sit in on *that* oncology meeting strikes me as selfish now. It was their son's life on the line.

A half hour passed after the nurses took my vitals and sent me back to the waiting room. Then forty-five minutes. Though I sat with a casual posture, my insides were coiling. I feared that my new oncologist was taking a long time because he was consulting with Dr. Luce because my PET-scan results showed that my cancer was active, and now he had to figure out how to break this terrible news to me (*bad news, buddy!*) and figure out a new plan of attack on my resilient lymphoma. But then another part of my mind came to the rescue. *Occam's razor! Occam's razor!* this voice of reason beckoned; the explanation for his delay was likely much simpler. Dr. Dean probably had some time-consuming, first-time meetings with other new patients like me.

Once the clock crept up to 10 a.m., just as I began to really freak out, Dr. Dean leaned in the doorway to call my name.

"I'm sorry I'm running a little behind today," he said, introducing himself with a handshake. He was tall with an athletic build and appeared to be in his mid-thirties. He sped down the hallway. I had to walk at a brisk pace to keep up with him as we sped past all the people standing in the hallway.

In the exam room, I took a seat beside his desk.

"How are you doing?" Dr. Dean asked, shuffling through pages in my file. He had a confident, charismatic voice. He sounded like the kind of guy who could pick up women at bars.

"I'm hanging in there," I said with an upbeat tone.

He paused, his eyes still focused on my paper work.

"Well, your PET scan looks good."

Those six words left me stunned. I waited for him to qualify his statement. We sat there quietly for a few seconds before I thought, *My god, that's it? THAT'S how you're going to tell me the sweetest news I have ever wanted to hear in my life?*

"The scan showed that there is no metastatic activity in the mediastinal area. The PET scan measures your body's metabolic activity—FDG avidity—and found no activity in your chest. There's still a small mass where the tumor used to be, but it continues to be metabolically suppressed. So, we can say that your disease is in remission."

My hands were clasped over my knees. I leaned forward and smiled back at him.

"Now we just need to figure out how to keep tracking you, since there *is* something physical—this little, tiny thing that we need to keep an eye on."

Dr. Dean proceeded to tell me that he had consulted with Dr. Luce. Since I had a small mass in my chest—which was likely scar tissue—he recommended that I get a chest x-ray done every four months. That way, we could see if it went away or grew—which would be bad with a capital "B." Blood tests would have to be done as well. I would always have to keep a vigilant eye out for any physical symptoms, namely swollen lymph nodes. I nodded, then asked if I could get a copy of the PET-scan report. It was going to be a million times better than those straight-A grade-school report cards my parents used to put up on the fridge.

As he filled out a blood lab form for my next checkup, I looked out the window behind him. Past the brick roof, a dark cover of clouds rolled by. Drizzle fell on the windowpane. Not exactly the sunlight I felt brimming inside, but I gave a dumb, contented grin as I looked at the floor by my feet. *This is it*—the moment I had dreamt of since that morning I awoke in my bedroom with the knowledge that I had a killer blooming inside my body. I could feel my eyes well up with tears, but I spared Dr. Dean of having to deal with that awkwardness. (What does a man do when he sees another grown man crying?) I knew they would probably spill later.

While he filled out another form, Dr. Dean filled the silence by asking me again how I was doing.

"Well, I feel great now," I said. "Relieved. I have a lot going on right now, but this was the main thing I was freaking out about."

Dr. Dean made a follow-up appointment in four months. We shook hands and left the exam room. I took my place in line to schedule my appointment with the receptionist. It kinda sucked to have to stand there and wait like a normal human being when inside I was bouncing like Tigger and shaking my arms and yelling like a kid who had just won a shopping spree at Toys "R" Us.

It was drizzling when I descended the front steps to Ward 86. I walked over to a side of the building to stand underneath a stairwell. I called my mom's extension at Cabrillo Elementary.

"This is Teresa," she said in her thick Spanish accent.

"Hi, Mom, it's me."

She made a slight gasp—the good kind. From the tone of my voice, she could tell what I had to say.

"¿Cómo estás, mi hijo?"

"Well, I just got out of my doctor's appointment—and I have some really good news. The cancer's gone. It's not active or growing anymore."

"Oh, that's great news, mi hijo."

I went on to explain everything that Dr. Dean had told me regarding the physical mass in my chest, the follow-up tests I would have to take, and that the mass would likely dissolve in time. She was choked up by the time I finished.

"This makes me very happy, Juanito."

I felt my throat choke up. Tears fell down my cheeks as I stepped out from beneath the stairwell to gaze up at the gray sky, smiling as the rain washed over me.

On the train ride to school later that day, Paola texted: "I gather that you are in remission? If so, congrats!" She must have found out via the Facebook posting I made earlier that day in which I shared the Good News with my cyber peeps. After all we had gone through during that crazy period of my life, I felt bad that this was the impersonal manner in which she found out. It didn't feel right. But, if she couldn't make the relationship commitment I had hoped for, then I was determined to be distant toward her.

I'm not sure what I thumbed back in response. It may have been a simple "Thanks!" or I may have thanked Paola and told her that she helped me through it. And I believe she did—with her love, her willingness to listen to my troubles. She was the one person who heard me complain about the mundane matters tied to my battle with lymphoma, such as the long lines at the hospital or the difficulty I encountered in obtaining my nausea medicine. She was my witness through that trying period of my life.

Once at the Orinda station, I bumped into Wesley at the bus stop. We sat in the back of the bus as it winded through the woodsy town. He told me that he was a little nervous about his literature class that afternoon. It was the first time his undergraduate class would discuss *Don Quixote*, which they were reading in its entirety. He was excited to talk about Cervantes, to discuss how modern—even postmodern—the sixteenth-century tome was. Since I had not read it, Wesley began to describe its metafictional quality, how the book is a "mortal combat" for the protagonists.

As the bus turned onto the driveway to campus, I said, "Speaking of mortal combats, I went to my oncologist today, and Mr. Hodgkins is dead."

Wesley's blue eyes opened wide, his mouth agape to let out an "*oooh!*"

"I got a PET scan done last week, and the cancer's gone."

"That's great news!" he said with a wry smile.

"It really is. I just don't know how to celebrate it, ya know? How do you celebrate something like this?"

"Are you still with Paola? I'm sorry, but Barbara told me she wasn't sure if you two were still together."

"It's cool. We're not. We finally broke up, for good." (Or so I thought then.)

"Oh, that's too bad," he said as the bus pulled up to its stop by the chapel, "because otherwise I'd say you two should drink some champagne and have some sex."

I roared as we stepped off the bus.

Later that evening, Paola sent a text in Spanish. She wrote, "I'm very happy that you've realized your dream. I hope your good health lasts. I wish you the very best." It pleased me to read, though I could sense she felt conflicted.

That night, my buddy Jonny invited me out for celebratory drinks in the Castro. At the bar, we exchanged hearty hugs. "Congratulations! This is such great news!" he said.

I smiled and thanked him. A big part of me didn't believe it was such great news. It's not like I was in the clear—and I wouldn't be for another five years, and then only *if* I remained in remission.

But if my one friend who was a cancer survivor thought it was great news, maybe it really was.

Yippee . . .

A WEEK AFTER I received the Good News, Rick, Mariana, our parents, and I went out for a celebratory lunch. It was late Monday morning at a pizza joint in Noe Valley. I sat in the curved leather booth at the head of our table. Lunch was Mariana's idea. I was grateful that she wanted to bring us together, but I would have rather stayed home. I slept like shit the night before. It had been over a week since I had a decent night of sleep. When I stared past our table to the sunlight streaming through the window, it was a humming white that made me squint. Even the coffee I guzzled could not kick-start my weary spirit.

The past week had been exhausting. School, work, and searching for a new home. Every day I spent at least an hour searching and respond-ing to Craigslist postings. I had visited two prospective households in the Mission. The first host mentioned "roommates" in his response but nothing about seven people sharing one small kitchen and two bath-rooms. The second place held an open house. A cocky, long-haired freelance graphic designer with a surfer voice held court upon a stool in the kitchen while a crowd of smiley applicants stood around to answer his questions. It felt like some icky game show: Who's Hip and Progressive Enough for Our Vacant Bedroom? And the past Saturday, Paola and I met for the first time since I broke up with her.

We had a writing date at Socha Café. We wanted to remain friends, to be supportive of each other's work. At the café, I even cracked jokes about how she didn't have to deal with me anymore. I was hopeful that we could exist more easily as friends someday. I told Paola that per-haps this was what was meant for us. I had just finished reading Evan Handler's memoir, *Time on Fire: My Comedy of Terrors*. He eventually broke up with the girlfriend who stuck with him during his harrowing battle with leukemia. They remained close friends, which was encouraging to read. That prospect didn't seem to inspire Paola, though. And she had no sense of humor about my jokes. She was still hurting.

From Socha Café, Paola and I walked seven long blocks to meet the rest of our writing group for dinner. We found it difficult to converse. The drone of passing cars became repugnant; they brought hyper-attention to the awkward silences between us, to our conversation, which was cordial and stilted like one between strangers on a plane. Weeks before, we had spoken freely and held hands when we walked down the street. Now there was a gaping gulf between us. It was difficult to witness what we had become.

At the restaurant, Rick and Mariana chirped and joked with my parents as we awaited our food. They were carefree, jovial. With my exhausted spirit, I found it difficult to feel happy like them. My good health was on its way to being restored—but for how long? I didn't know. None of us did. Besides the toll the treatment had inflicted on my body, effects I did not know then, the battle for my life had come at a steep price. I had lost Paola. My best friend. (I am not delusional enough to believe that our relationship would have lasted if I never had lymphoma, but I am certain it would have been easier on us. My problems with alcohol, anger, and the criticisms I made during our relationship were matters I was solely culpable of. But without all that darkness, without all that anger, Paola and I may have had a better shot. That's what I believed then.)

Once our food was served, Rick raised his cup of water.

"Cheers! ¡Salud, salud!" he said, looking at me. I managed a half grin and clanged my coffee mug with their glasses. I thanked them for coming out.

Our toast made me even sadder. Somewhere inside I was happy for them, happy my parents were chipper instead of glum like they often were during my infusions. While I watched my family, all smiles, I realized how alone I was. They could not understand what I was going through. They could not understand that these fears I had over cancer would likely never end. They could not understand that those dark ominous clouds that had hovered over me during the past year and a half had not blown away; they had only rolled further off, up into the sky—but they could come back. They could not understand how scared

I felt at the thought of those dark clouds returning. I was not sure if I would have the will to go through that struggle again. I imagined I would be so appalled to be struck twice with cancer when I knew a number of people who lived much unhealthier lives, such as an ex-roommate who smoked cigarettes for breakfast and drank like a fish, or Rick who was an alcoholic and ate poorly. If cancer returned for a sequel, I was afraid I would crumble to my knees, profoundly wail, then wipe the tears from my eyes to glower up at the sky and say, "Fuck it. I. Am. Done."

When I realized how alone I was among my own family, I had an aha moment: my parents and sisters were the audience for this book. In our creative writing classes, we had discussed "our reader(s)" a number of times. Since it was unreasonable to expect that everyone could or would want to *get* what we were individually writing, our professors suggested that it might be helpful to envision someone, or a group of people, to write to.

But first and foremost, this book has always been for me. Writing it has been instrumental in figuring out how I feel about what happened to me, in figuring out who I wanted to be in the aftermath of my strug-gle—and in figuring out who I no longer wanted to be. Writing this memoir has been the most challenging and loving act I have given myself.

That afternoon, I felt a glimmer of solace infuse me. If I wrote this book so I would never have to explain any part of this journey to my family, then I had fulfilled my duty. By recognizing, then accepting, the loneliness cancer had brought, something shifted within me.

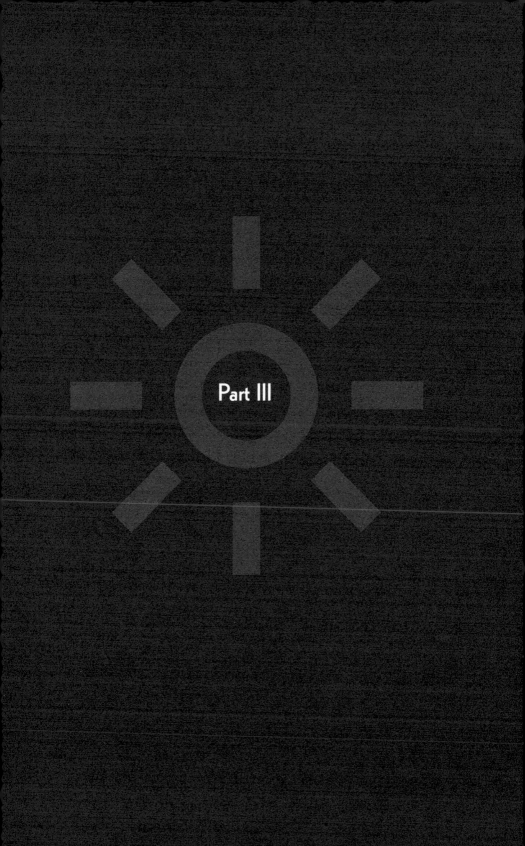

Part III

¡March Locura!

THERE I WAS, on the morning of the vernal equinox, pedaling on an exercise bike at my gym, watching the final minutes of the Saint Mary's men's basketball game against the second-seeded Villanova Wildcats. One minute and thirty-five seconds remained on the clock. It was a tie game, 65–65, after Villanova's point guard made two crucial free throws. By then, I had been on the exercise bike for over an hour. My tank top was drenched in sweat. I could have wrung out a cup of sweat, I swear.

On the ensuing possession, the ball was inbounded to Mickey McConnell, our sharp-shooting junior guard who had made two three-point bombs in the opening minutes of the game in which the ball rainbowed through the rim like a mesmerizing trick shot. Once he passed half court, McConnell dribbled left, trying to shake his defender with a high post pick from Omar Samhan, our 6'11" star center who had played the game of his life, scoring thirty-two points on the biggest stage. His defender stuck to him—that is, until McConnell did a cross-over to free himself behind the three-point line. He spotted up and launched an arcing twenty-five-foot shot that prompted one of the announcers to say, "Wow," and then both announcers shouted "Ohhh-hhh!" along with the thundering crowd when the ball banked high off the glass and into the basket to give the tenth-seeded Gaels an improb-able 68–65 lead with a minute and fifteen seconds left. My eyes popped and I shouted, "Whoaaaaa!" as the Saint Mary's bench players leaped from their seats, hugging one another with unabashed glee as Villanova called a time out. Minutes later, after McConnell and Matthew Della-vedova went a cold-blooded six-for-six from the free throw line, Saint

Mary's advanced to the Sweet Sixteen round of the NCAA Men's Basketball Tournament for the first time. It was the biggest win in school history.

Once the game was over, I hopped off the exercise bike. I hooted, clapping with a mile-wide grin on my face. A few other gym patrons hooted and clapped. With my hand towel wrapped around my neck, I triumphantly marched into the locker room.

And that moment encapsulates what Life after Lymphoma felt like after that gloomy celebratory lunch with my family.

In all, it felt like a grand curtain had been parted to allow a pileup of delirious goodness to brighten all the facets of my life. At school, our campus was abuzz from our basketball team's performance in the collegiate tournament. My writing was coming along. Marilyn, my ever-generous mentor, loved the revised first chapter of the memoir, as did my workshop class. I was no longer upset about having to move out; it's not like I had any control over that decision. To boot, the late winter days were becoming sunnier and sunnier. Led Zeppelin's godly "Kashmir" was the song I felt thumping in my heart throughout the middle part of March, especially its opening verse. Paola and I even reconciled. During the early morning hours of the first day of spring, Paola curled beside me, resting her head over my chest. A shoulder-high pile of empty boxes stood at the foot of my bed. My bookshelves and CD towers were emptied. While I held Paola, I stared at my bamboo blinds. Together we saw the dark sky gently trickle with light. It was the first time we saw the sunrise.

Later that day, I was offered a room in the Mission I had interviewed for. I was giddy and relieved. My search for a new home had been exhausting. The new place was not a beautiful home like Casa 909. Its surrounding neighborhood wasn't as great, either, but at least I was staying in the neighborhood. Though it would be many months before I confessed it to Paola, one of the reasons I wanted to stay in the Mission was so I could be close to her.

Although I was wary about getting back with her, it felt like something *had* changed between us. It was as if we were lighter, no longer burdened by our tumultuous past. But I had overlooked that her family *still* hated me. This had already become such a detrimental factor in our relationship.

Now I believe that the change I felt between us was mostly within me. The sheer happiness I felt in the afterglow of the Good News made most of March a crazy-wonderful ride. Even in therapy, I was full of smiles and quips that managed to crack Akhila's serious-therapist demeanor a number of times. "I'm happy to have problems," I told her during one of our sessions. "It sure beats being dead." I could have attracted a swarm of moths with the brightness I exuded then. And the difference was this: for the first time in my life, I grasped how wonderful and deliriously joyous it is to simply be alive and healthy. If cancer survivorship teaches anything, it is that. And it's a gift that keeps giving, a ride that never gets old—*if* you remember.

In the infancy of my Life after Lymphoma, I had come to accept—even embrace—the flux of change swirling around me. As hippie as it may sound, there was nothing I could do but try to make the best of what the present gave me.

So Long, 909

A FEW DAYS before I moved out of Casa 909, I sat cross-legged in the middle of the living room. I was watching an old *Simpsons* episode. Before me, serving as a culinary altar, was an upturned bucket. Atop it rested a greasy burrito, which I poured green salsa over. The room was nearly empty. Gone were the brown chairs and the green couch I used to love to read from—the same couch I sat on when I discovered two swollen lymph nodes. Gone was the modest wooden table that supported its share of wine glasses and delectable treats over the years from our dinner parties. Gone were Amber's paintings of Django Reinhardt, Louis Armstrong, and her haunting self-portrait in which she sung behind a vintage microphone with an abnormally elongated neck and mouth that was reminiscent of Edvard Munch's *The Scream*. Gone were our communal books and DVDs that used to rest on the shelves. No one was home. Kelly's room was practically empty. Ditto for Crystal. I stuffed my mouth with the burrito and tortilla chips and cackled like a hyena at Homer's harebrained antics. With the absence of paintings and furniture, my laughter echoed off the walls, filling the empty flat.

Someone came through the front door, then ascended the stairs. The footsteps continued down the hallway. After living with Amber for over three years, I recognized the cadence of her walk. She passed by the living room, a paper bag in hand. She nodded approvingly at my lunch and entertainment selections before we greeted each other. I told her I cleaned the moldy ceiling of our bathroom as best as I could. A pungent whiff of bleach hung in the hallway. Despite a few washings, my hands still had a sterile, bleachy smell reminiscent of hospitals.

The morning I moved out, after a day and night of exhaustive cleaning, Amber and I said good-bye outside her bedroom. Mom was sweeping my vacant bedroom. Dad was carrying a few of my light belongings down to the moving truck outside. A laborer we picked up by the U-Haul was chilling outside, drinking a bottle of juice my mom brought. I handed Amber my house key. She thanked me for all of my help in cleaning. I brushed it off, saying it was the least I could do. It was the last time I could show my love to that house. We hugged and wished each other well.

Before I closed the front door one last time, I walked upstairs. I scanned my empty room before I strode over to the kitchen—the first part of the flat I was shown when I interviewed for the vacant room. Standing there rekindled a memory from the housewarming party my roommates threw for me and another roomie who had moved in. Mariana and Rick, Judy and Carlisle were there. They loved my new home, especially the cozy kitchen. Leaning against the kitchen doorway, wine glass in hand, Judy said it was the kind of place to live at before I moved out on my own for good, or with a significant other. I smiled when she said that. "You're right!" I said, my friends and loved ones huddled around me. And I hoped she was. Back then, I was in a relationship with Julia. Life didn't pan out between us like I had hoped. I was leaving Casa 909 to move into another household with three roommates. But it had been a good home.

A few months into chemotherapy, I talked to Paola and my roomies and friends about moving out of San Francisco. I would never forget that my body developed cancer in that city. Sometimes when I cycled around the Mission, inhaling exhaust from cars while waiting at a signal, I would get distressed. My mind would motor, *You've got to get out of here. You've GOT to get out of here. This city life is unhealthy for you.* Casa 909 came to have similar cancerous associations. That's why a part of me was relieved to leave it behind, despite the fact that I knew that living in that charming Victorian house, built in 1912, had nothing to do with developing a rare blood cancer.

Nowadays, on the occasions I have walked or ridden past Casa 909, I usually sigh. *Ah, the old neighborhood*, I say to myself or to whomever I am riding with. Good ol' Mama's Market. Bubbles Laundromat. The nonnative palm trees lining Dolores Street that nevertheless seem to fit. The school across the street from our home, which often roared with the shouts of children whenever the school bell rang. The steep hill to Dolores Park, the one I cycled over and zipped down for my radiation treatments. The picturesque view of the Mission District from the corner of 21st and Ames Streets with Potrero Hill in the distance. And the tranquil block of Fair Oaks Street between 21st and 22nd Streets, which I loved to stroll on my way home.

On that block, there are two trees beside the Laundromat that I was fond of; they looked like lovers, their branches intertwined, as if they were embracing. During my nighttime strolls home, from time to time—once I checked to see that no one was around—I would wrap my arms around one of the trees. Taking a deep breath, I would embrace it, my cheek against its bark. I was always aware that I should have never been embarrassed to hug that tree (or any, really), but I didn't want my neighbors to think I was cuckoo.

One breezy evening, I came upon those trees. I think it was a few days after Paola's twenty-eighth birthday, maybe a few days after our trip to Seattle. I was very down on myself. Weighed down with guilt, awash in regret. When I came to one of the trees, I realized that it was time to begin to lift my head, time to let go of that oppressive shame. I wrapped my arms around it and nestled my face against its trunk.

It's a lesson I am still trying to learn.

Let the Reconstruction Begin

One does not become enlightened by imagining figures of light, but by making the darkness conscious. The latter procedure, however, is disagreeable and therefore not popular.

—CARL JUNG, *The Collected Works of C. G. Jung, Volume 13: Alchemical Studies*, 1968

ONE SUNNY WEEKDAY, a few weeks before my thirty-first birthday,[*] I marched out of the house wearing shorts and flip-flops. In my bag, I carried a towel and a spiral notebook. Dolores Park was my destination. I had given myself a difficult writing mission: to jot down the memories that ashamed me the most—the worst acts I had done while drunk.

At the sun-drenched park, I set my towel on a hill that overlooked the urban oasis, faced Mission High School's picturesque bell tower. In the distance, the jungle of skyscrapers sprawled out before my eyes.

---

[*] My first postcancer birthday snuck up on me since I was über-busy with school, work, and my move. Once I realized its significance, I hesitated to make plans. The only certainty was that I did *not* want to have a big drunken party like the year before.

In the end, my family and I convened for a dinner at Rick and Mariana's house on a dreary, rainy April afternoon in San Francisco. Though I am grateful to have had a dinner with my family, my thirty-first birthday has been allotted to the crummy column in my mind because I had invited some supposedly good friends, a handful of classmates, and my writing group posse, but only my friend Andy showed up. That was disappointing enough, but what made me downright pissed off was that most of them didn't even respond to the Facebook invitation I had sent a week before my birthday. How difficult is it to say no, type a short response, then click "Reply"? I felt hurt, confounded. Their nonresponses to my invitation made me question those friendships.

Ultimately, my thirty-first birthday taught me that I no longer liked to celebrate my birthdays with a group of people. I didn't like the expectations I built of such celebrations, the subsequent expectations I made of others. My birthdays have always been a big deal to me, but I was far less apt to get disappointed if I just celebrated them on my own, coupled with a tranquil home-cooked dinner with my parents, the two people I owe everything to.

Past the downtown skyline, the Bay Bridge could be seen. I took off my shirt and sat cross-legged on top of my towel amid a scattering of sunbathers. A few dogs ran about, chasing the balls their young owners tossed. Pencil in hand, iPod by my side, I flipped the notebook to a few blank pages. I stared off, thinking of those moments I was haunted by. I dove in and began to write them down.

The sunshine and the jovial, relaxed spirit around me was a stark contrast to the dread and shame I felt as I reimagined those memories. Like the time I slapped my mother upside the head in front of an aunt because she mistakenly thought my girlfriend's eyes were blue instead of hazel. Or the car accident I had when I was twenty-one, somber and loaded on a sixer of Mickey's, my girlfriend and my friend riding in the car while we dropped off our buddy Johnny at the Amtrak station in San José so he could live with his family in East L.A. since his life had spiraled into a sad rut. My blackout at Oktoberfest. My twenty-seventh birthday when I broke my girlfriend's windshield with a brick. And so on, and so on. Reliving those memories was like standing alone on a beach and raising my hands higher and higher to conjure a tidal wave of guilt, shame, and regret to pummel me.

I left Dolores Park—aptly named that day—hiding behind my pair of aviators. My notebook had two pages full of small, neat handwriting. I went home and took those notes to write a crappy thirteen-page draft. That draft had its share of long footnotes where I essentially hid some of the memories I didn't want out in the body of the main text. Writing about alcohol-drenched moments—even ones that were painful to linger on—made me crave a cool beer. While I cranked out the first draft the rest of the day and night, I drank two bottles of beer. They were my reward for dredging through all that shit. That chapter was the most difficult thing I ever wrote.

Our nonfiction workshop teacher during that final semester at Saint Mary's was Jane Vandenburgh. She was a trip—a caring, amusing, kooky-grandmother type with a heap of youthful gusto. She had written a memoir about her troubled childhood—her father had committed suicide when she was nine, then her mother got committed to a mental hospital a few years later. Somehow, Jane survived her childhood, wrote several books, and thrived when so many others would have drowned from the life she was dealt. I had taken to heart one of the truths she told us throughout the semester—that if you write about difficult things you have done or been put through, the writing would allow you to let it go. Create emotional distance from that real-life content. Make it seem as if that person you are writing about is no longer *you*. The writing would allow you to *own* that difficult personal history. Jane made it seem as if it were a borderline magical process, one that helped to save her. I desperately wanted to believe that she was right—that I could begin to let go of the self-destructive spirit within me if I unflinchingly wrote about it.

I submitted that chapter to our workshop class. Jane commended my bravery in writing about those painful memories. She could relate to what I wrote. She had her own bout with alcoholism. She called me out on being a type of alcoholic when I was reluctant to admit it then.

Jane was right about the power of memoir writing. Those memories—like any we choose to remember—had done their part to *define* who I was. But within weeks of writing, sharing, and revising that chapter, I was able to casually tell my friends—even strangers—about some of those fucked-up things I had done. Prior to writing about them, some of those shame-filled memories had only been shared with a handful of my close friends. In no time, I found myself kidding about my skeletons in a self-deprecating way. To give an example, during a conversation with Tagi that somehow or another turned to the subject of prostitutes, I said, "You better keep me away from them!" By choosing not to hide those memories inside anymore, they were deflated of the power I had given them.

It *was* almost magical how something shifted within me once I wrote about my skeletons and shared them with my classmates. I felt freed of much of the guilt, shame, and regret I had carried all those years.

On a bus ride to school, I jotted down a list of truths I had concluded about my relationship with alcohol. During a recent therapy session with Akhila, I had talked about my booziest moments. While I rehashed some incidents I had over the years, I was flabbergasted when she pointed out that I spoke about alcohol as if I were in a relationship with it. And Akhila was right. It *was* like a relationship. A troublesome, up-and-down one throughout my adulthood.

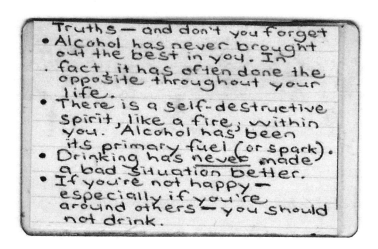

Truths — and don't you forget
• Alcohol has never brought
  out the best in you. In
  fact, it has often done the
  opposite throughout your
  life.
• There is a self-destructive
  spirit, like a fire, within
  you. Alcohol has been
  its primary fuel (or spark).
• Drinking has never made
  a bad situation better.
• If you're not happy —
  especially if you're
  around others — you should
  not drink.

Here's what I wrote on a 2" × 3" blank card:

I laminated the card. I have kept it tucked inside my wallet. It is with me wherever I go in case I have ever felt the need to remind myself. But thankfully, I have rarely had to. Those truths have been mostly internalized. I remember them like I remember that I had lymphoma.

And thankfully, the desire to drink excessively hardly happens now. It's as if it blew out of me.

The Freak Show

It's an insane world, and I'm proud to be a part of it.

—BILL HICKS, *Relentless*, 1992

IN OUR FREEWHEELING, hour-long sessions, in the sanctuary Akhila provided, I often talked about my memoir. Sitting in our armchairs, we would discuss something minute like a footnote or a single sentence. I was immersed in my work. Consumed by it as though I were submerged in its roiling water. Marilyn and I were meticulously revising it so I could submit a clean thesis manuscript. With Akhila, I talked about my book as if it were a living being.

I talked about Mr. Hodgkins, too. One of the first things I did in therapy was to describe him to Akhila in the way I had written about him. I felt it was important for her to be familiar with him, to see the daemon figure I had created. During one of our sessions, I told her, "It's a wonder I've never had a dream about Mr. Hodgkins—at least that I can remember." She seemed to dig it all. It was hard to know with certainty because I could never tell how much of her reactions were part of a psychotherapist act versus what was unfiltered (though I always suspected it was tilted toward the latter).

With time, Akhila harnessed this tendency of mine—to use analogies and symbols—to talk about my light and dark sides. When we discussed the chapter about my self-destructive spirit, we discussed those pained memories at length; she dubbed my dark side "El Diablito." I laughed. It was perfect. In turn, I called my good, repented side "San Juanito." This sober santito was the one who tiptoed onstage the morning after a drunken night to begin to clean up El Diablito's destructive mess. San Juanito was the good boy who had perfected the art of an anguished, shame-ridden apology.

In discussing my self-destructive behavior, Akhila and I discussed the larger world I saw. I mentioned the war, hate, exploitation, and destruction of the land we humans perpetuate for greed, wealth, consumption, and power. I thought of the unsustainable civilizations we build, the default suburban sprawl we continue to create for our American landscape. As far as I'm concerned, our supposedly civilized world is a deranged construct. Humanity seems self-destructive to me, like a devastating virus for our planet.* For years, it sickened and deeply saddened me to see and read about the seemingly never-ending destruction we have wrought as a species. (John Steinbeck once wrote, "I wonder why progress looks so much like destruction.") From time to time, I hit the bottle hard, thinking, *Why the fuck not?* Our lives are pointless because we're destroying ourselves and life on this planet. And not enough people seem to genuinely care.

Since it's impossible for me not to care about the well-being of our world, I concluded in therapy that the profound sadness, the subsequent anger I feel will *always* be inside me—however long I live. I have no hope that we will ever profoundly change, but I could no longer take humanity's self-destructiveness personally. Not anymore. I am responsible for my own shit, not everyone else's. With Akhila's help, I decided that was one of the paramount changes I needed in my rebirth. There is little I can do to change the world in a positive way, but I can change how I react to it.

The ship's going down for many life-forms on this planet—certainly on our way of living. I believe the gas pumps will rust someday. Our smoothly paved streets and highways will become cracked and desolate. Weeds and plant life will overrun them in time, finding root in their faults. (For a thorough and vivid description of all of this, check out Alan Weisman's *The World Without Us*.) Our landscape and coastlines will change as the polar shelves continue to break off and melt into the ocean. Our Mother Earth may wipe us humans out before we ever do so ourselves with deadly mutated viruses we will find no remedy for.

---

* "Every mammal on this planet instinctively develops a natural equilibrium with the surrounding environment, but you humans do not. You move to an area and you multiply and multiply until every natural resource is consumed and the only way you can survive is to spread to another area. There is another organism on this planet that follows the same pattern. Do you know what it is? A virus. Human beings are a disease, a cancer of this planet."—Agent Smith to Morpheus in the Wachowskis' classic *The Matrix*.

I do think our stint on this planet is accelerating to an end, but I am happy to be a tiny cell of this grandiose organism we call Planet Earth. (British philosopher and Buddhist Alan Watts once likened our planet to a "tremendous brain" in which every single being is but a cell, or an interconnected neuron.) I am pleased to be an insignificant yet interconnected little part of it in a way I never was before my corporeal vessel housed a deathly visitor. For the most part, I am thrilled to still be a part of "the freak show," as George Carlin put it. ("When you're born, you get a ticket to the *freak show*. When you're born in America, you get a front row seat.") I adore every single one of my gray hairs— my battle scars, my tree rings—that eventually sprouted once my hair grew back.

Life is hard, but I hope to have a head full of gray hairs someday.

Much Too Late

ON MAY 14, the day I defended my 132-page thesis before Marilyn and Wesley, Paola called me from Arizona. She and her sister had flown there to attend a wedding. I was in my bedroom while my roommates were out. As we continued chatting, it became apparent that she was upset about something. I asked what was wrong, but she wouldn't tell me. This went on for some time until I asked if it concerned our relationship. She told me it did but refused to elaborate.

"Paola, I think it's unfair of you to not discuss what is wrong since it affects *our* relationship," I said.

She sighed.

"I just got into a huge fight with my sister," she said. "We were talking when I made a mention of you. She asked what I was doing, hanging around with you, and I told her we were still seeing each other. And that's when she started yelling at me."

Paola was already receiving this pointed criticism from her mother. Now her older sister—who had been through the divorce ringer—was ragging on our relationship. On prior occasions, Rosa had warned Paola that the biggest mistake she made in her marriage was to put her faith in what her husband *could* be versus who he *was*. She had cautioned her sister to not make the same mistake.

Paola sounded beat. Drained. Hopeless. By that juncture in our seesaw relationship, the majority of our difficulties were tied to her family's incessant criticism of us. Paola was tremendously affected by what her family thought of her, especially her domineering mother. And sadly, her family was the kind of familial unit that believed that criticizing one another was the most exemplary way of demonstrating their love for one another. Paola was just like her siblings when she didn't like whomever they dated. On two occasions, she told me she got drunk and berated Jesús for dating an older woman she did not approve of. It was a vicious, critical, judgmental cycle they must have adopted from their unaffectionate Catholic mother, who probably learned it from her God-fearing, old-school-traditional Mexican family.

With that phone call, it began to dawn on me just how devastating her family's opinion of me was going to be on our relationship. That mess I left in Seattle—by not apologizing to Jesús for the way I treated Paola that first night—had formed into a mountain of trouble.

"Paola, *I need* to try to make things better between me and your family," I said. "After I'm done with school, what if I flew to Seattle to begin to patch things up with your siblings?"

She was silent on her end. Meanwhile—in what strikes me now as symbolic—I was perched up on my dresser, beside my window. For much of our conversation, I half-stood on it, bending toward the ceiling since it was the best way to get any reception in our house.

"What if I reach out to Rosa and Jesús through Facebook—send them messages asking for their forgiveness? To explain my actions during our trip to Seattle? What if I ask them, without saying it, to leave us be so we can continue to try to make our relationship a healthier one?"

"It's no use," Paola said. "They're too stubborn. Too thickheaded to hear you out."

"You're probably right, but we can *at least* try. I really don't think we have anything to lose."

Paola sighed.

Then she told me something that should have deterred me from reaching out to her siblings: she found out that Rosa and Jesús knew I was sick when we visited them. Shortly after I was diagnosed, Paola told her mother, who in turn told them. It flustered me to hear this. During our trip, neither one of her siblings reached out to me. Never asked how I was doing. Never attempted to become personally acquainted with me in any significant way, though I never did either.

But I was desperate to make amends with her family. I felt so culpable for all the missteps I had made since that fateful trip, especially the bad impression I must have made when Rosa visited the year before, and all the time that elapsed without an apology from me. Months before Paola made that call from Arizona, I thought about sending her mother and siblings cards to apologize for my actions, but then I broke up with Paola in late February; it was pointless to reach out to her siblings if we didn't even have a commitment to stand on together. When I reflected on all those missed opportunities, I couldn't help but feel like maybe we were simply not meant to be together.

Despite this, I wasn't ready to give up on Paola. Not when things between us were beginning to feel easy again, when it seemed like we were building a new foundation that a healthy relationship could grow from. In our short time together, we had endured too much to cave in from negative influences outside of our relationship.

Once we hung up, I sat on my lounge chair and composed two long messages on my laptop. When I clicked the "send" button on the second message (one to Jesús), I knew what I had done was futile. Those messages would not accomplish what I hoped for. As though I had become an omniscient being, I saw myself sitting in that chair, facing the window, sending apologetic messages to people I hardly knew. This is not what happens to maintain a healthy, lasting relationship, I thought. In my heart, I knew our relationship was done.

I texted Paola to tell her I sent the messages. She texted back that she appreciated it. She also told me she had some family issues that needed to be addressed if she ever wanted to have a good relationship. She was going to seek therapy. It was up to me if I wanted to continue to try and work things out between us. Since she forgave me on a few occasions, I felt it was only right to demonstrate faith and patience with her, even though I felt emotionally pummeled.

As expected, Rosa's and Jesus's responses were harsh. Reading them was like getting socked in the gut. In his message, Jesús questioned my apology. He asked why I was, after all this time, suddenly feeling bad about my actions in Seattle. He thought I wrote my apology only so I could tell Paola that I tried to patch things up with them. He also wrote that he didn't know me and didn't care to try to know me, which was the gist of his entire response. Rosa was equally dismissive but in a terse, diplomatic fashion (with much better grammar and punctuation, might I add). She rightly told me that my actions were disrespectful to her family. Later, she wrote that it didn't matter to her if I felt sorry for my actions, nor did she pretend to know what I had gone through or what I was trying to do to change my life. She closed by wishing me good luck, which was her gentle, veiled way of saying "piss off."

317

In the messages I sent to Paola's siblings, I went to lengths to explain where I was, physically and mentally, that Thursday night in Seattle. I did not blame my illness for my actions, but I had asked for *some* empathy from them. I asked for the possibility of forgiveness down the road. Deep down, I *wanted* them to forgive me, like the devout Catholics they purported to be. But instead they were cold, unforgiving, and heartless to me, as well as to their sister: unwilling to listen to Paola when she told them I was growing into a better partner. They seemed accustomed to talking down to their little sister instead of genuinely listening to her.

If Paola and I had any sense, we would have ended our relationship, once and for all, after her siblings carved their verdict of me. But we genuinely loved each other. That always seemed to be our problem (and I said this to her on several occasions). By that point, I believe I had come to love and accept Paola more for who she was versus who I wanted her to be when I first fell for her. I did not criticize her as much as I had earlier. Slowly, I was learning that criticizing loved ones rarely accomplished any good. Instead of parting ways, Paola and I continued to follow love's senseless cadence. (My eyes went more and more astray, though, searching for someone new. A blank page to begin with.) Four months later, I broke up with her for good, though we would still—on occasion—mess around, then hang out in our old familiar way.

The primary reason for my decision to break up with her was because of her family. Once I fucked up, it seemed like they would never be wiling to forgive me. Months later, Paola's mother threatened to cancel a visit to San Francisco if it meant having dinner with me at some point. Her family's opinion of me was formed and that was that. Finito. End of discussion. Through their words and actions, I understood that they would never accept me. Good lord, they would have *really* detested me if they ever found out I was an atheist. (Paola never told her family about my spiritual beliefs. Once we began dating, she only mentioned to her mother that I had been raised Catholic.)

Since Paola wanted her family to be a significant part of her life, down life's road, I could not warm to the idea of having her toxic, judgmental, close-minded family as part of mine. My family was *not* like them. We were far more laid-back, affectionate, and compassionate. I couldn't see both families fitting together.

For me, leaving Paola because of her family was an act of self-love. I knew I was a better person than they imagined me to be. And I deserved better than them.

The week leading up to my graduation, I visited the Andy Warhol exhibit on campus that Wesley curated. Along the exhibit walls, in large lettering, were a few of Warhol's sterling quotes. One read: "It's not what you are that counts; it's what they think you are."

So true, I lamented. So very, very true.

Graduation

DONNING A BLACK robe and graduate cap, I walked single file into McKeon Pavilion with my fellow graduating classmates. The gymnasium floor was covered with the dark-gray butcher paper I had seen at last year's graduation. This time, the rows of empty folding chairs were waiting to be filled by us.

Our loved ones sat in the bleachers, snapping pictures while "Pomp and Circumstance" filled the gym with its grace. After we marched down the center aisle and filed into our section, I looked up into the stands where Carmen had texted to tell me where they sat. I smiled and waved when I saw Carmen, Rick, Mariana, Paola, and my parents waving to me. I blew kisses to them and took my seat beside Gaby—a jovial poet who wrote prose that made me gasp in awe. We sat at the end of our row beside the center aisle, next to the poets and Fictionistas.

By then, my cheeks were physically strained from all the grinning I had done backstage. (I didn't know it was possible to strain your cheek muscles from excessive smiling!) In a gymnasium hallway, our department chatted it up, complimenting one another on how spiffy and cute we looked. Decked out in a scholarly black robe, Marilyn brimmed with excitement as well. I had never seen her that bright and happy. We were a supremely excited bunch—all those books we devoured, all those classroom discussions, all those manuscripts we critiqued, and all those nights we stayed up writing had culminated into that singular moment.

Throughout the ceremony, I made quips to Gaby. Bless her, she was a receptive audience. Once the commencement speaker took the podium to deliver a predictable speech, we whispered about our respective postgraduation plans. It was the question everyone and their mother had been asking us for the weeks and months leading up to graduation: "What are you going to do after you graduate?" Gaby talked about moving in with her partner, about continuing to work a catering job that allowed her lots of time to read and write. I talked about applying for artist residencies. I told her my main postgraduate concern was falling back into a life-sucking nine-to-five existence that I had done for years before I returned to school. Too often, that kind of life didn't provide enough time for my writing. And I knew that's what I needed to keep me happy in postgraduate life. It was good to share this with someone who understood.

After the commencement speaker finished his speech, the stage behind him filled with our professors. One by one, the department heads stepped up to the podium to call up their graduates. School by school, graduate after graduate was summoned to receive their diploma. The gymnasium filled with applause, shouts, and an occasional peculiar hoot that made us all laugh.

Then Marilyn walked up to the podium. Our creative writing department stood. We walked over to the right side of the gym. I waved to my loved ones in the stands as we inched toward the stage in a single line. As I heard my classmates' names and the subsequent applause, I kept thinking, *Don't trip on the steps, don't trip on the steps!* That was followed by a thought stream of, *Left hand diploma, right hand shake, left hand diploma, right hand shake.* Before I knew it, it was my turn to step up to the stage. Shaking hands with Marilyn and our school president was a wide-eyed blur (though somehow or another I *did* fumble the diploma-handshake exchange). I stepped off the stage over to Wesley, who stood to the side. We embraced and nearly butted our foreheads before I turned my back to him so he could flip over our department's magenta-and-blue sash. I tried too hard to remember what he would say, imprint it in my memory along with the surge of emotions I felt, though I think he simply said, "Congratulations. You were great." I walked back to my seat, holding my head high like I had been knighted.

Being the sentimental yearner that I am, I figured I would cry the sweetest tears of joy I had ever felt in my life at some point during the ceremony. There was no ceremony when I finished chemotherapy, or when I was told that my disease was in remission. Graduating from Saint

Mary's was all of that rolled into returning to the non-graduate-school world as a changed man. I had been tested like I never had been before. Along the way, I discovered an inner resolve that I never knew I had.

The only time I felt shook up was when our school president, Brother Gallagher, closed the ceremony. He asked the crowd to outstretch their hands toward us graduates. He asked our loved ones to wish us well as we set forth to do good with the knowledge we had been graced with. While the crowd held out their hands toward us, I stood with my hands clasped behind my back, bowing my head.

Those two years at graduate school affirmed that writing was the best part of me. My hospital caregivers had provided my physical salvation, but I contained my spiritual redemption. My two-year journey through school while battling lymphoma taught me that I wouldn't want to live if I couldn't write—if I couldn't create, if I couldn't help others with their writing. I live to write; I write to live. It is that simple.

Standing in front of my chair, watching the commencement come to an end, I was not sure where life—however much I had left—would take me. None of us knew. I held that ceremonial diploma knowing only that *I had* to craft a life immersed with words, stories, manuscripts full of marginalia, and other fellow writers who burned with the same need. It was the truest way I could honor all the extra breaths I had been gifted.

In the photos my family took after the ceremony outside McKeon Pavilion, posing with mis papas, mis hermanas, then with Paola amid a sea of graduates and their loved ones, I looked really darn happy. Photo after photo, I beamed as though I were a pro at this whole smiling-on-cue deal. But that's not the case. Far from it, actually. Ever since I was a boy, I have disliked smiling for pictures. Instead, I would goofily cross my eyes, or make weird faces, or sigh and pout for the single frozen frame. Within my family, I became infamous for those poses. According to my mom, I "ruined" many a family picture. To this day, I still feel this dastardly impulse to make a goofy face rather than smile for pictures like some happy machine, but on my graduation from Saint Mary's, I couldn't get enough of the picture-taking. I hammed it up with the balloons my sisters gave me, with any of my loved ones. I was an insatiable photography subject that afternoon. Shit, if Dick Cheney were in attendance, I was liable to throw my arm around him and smile big for the camera.

Ever since I "beat cancer," I've noticed that I'm more willing to smile for pictures. My issue with grinning for pictures was always that I didn't want to smile unless I felt genuinely happy in that moment. (Plus, I don't have George Hamilton teeth.) But now I find it easier to summon enough sincere gratitude and happiness to produce a manufactured smile.

I am alive and well, after all.

Back home in Fremont, Paola and I sat beside each other on the couch, surrounded by my family. Instead of going out to a semi-fancy restaurant in Lafayette like I really kinda wanted, I asked that we order some pizzas back home so my tío José Luis, cousin Juan Luis, and Heide could more easily join in our festivities.

Weeks later, Paola told me she had never seen me happier.

And it's true.

I had never felt so proud of myself.

A Moment with Negrita

NEGRITA WAS ASLEEP on my parents' couch, curled up on an alpaca blanket. I sat at the dining table, writing on my laptop. It was well past midnight. The living room lamp was on, providing diffused light I hoped was not too bright for her. Once I realized it was one in the morning, I walked around the couch. "Negris," I said, leaning over her. "Sweetie, I'm sorry but I have to take you out to your bed." I gently reached beneath her to lift and cradle her against my chest.

The garage was pitch dark and colder than our heated home. I would have felt bad if I turned on the light, considering how blaringly bright it would be to her sleepy eyes. Instead, I gingerly stepped along the front bumper of my mother's car, nudging into it with the side of my leg. Like this, I eased my way to the stack of boxes where Negrita's bed rested. It was faintly lit by the streetlight outside the window that looked out onto our front lawn.

I lifted Negrita onto the yellow blanket atop the stack of boxes. I watched her shadowy outline as she walked about, silhouetted by the soft light behind her. "I'm sorry, kitty, but you have to sleep out here," I whispered, leaning my face toward her. Negrita stepped forward to nuzzle my forehead. When I leaned back to pet Negrita, I noticed the pale moonlight falling on her. The lawn behind her was brushed with a milky luminescence. All I could hear was the soft purring hum from her chest.

As I petted Negrita, my eyes began to well up. I knew she would die someday, and I just might be around to witness it—to see her still corpse, her closed eyes, with no purring emanating from her chest. I might grow old with her.

"I love you, kitty," I said, kissing the top of her head. Then I walked back into the house to wake for another day.

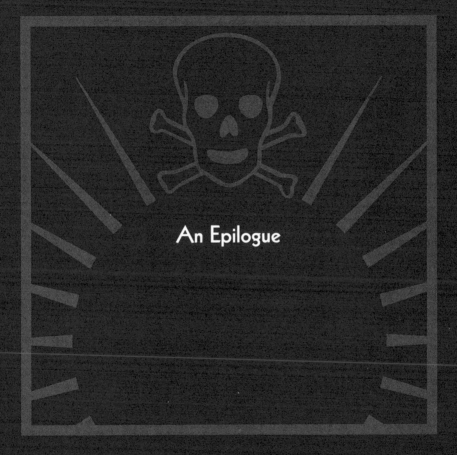

An Epilogue

THERE I WAS, back at the Mt. Zion lobby, shoulder bag slung over my black pea coat. It was June 10, 2010. I was there to visit David. He had called me earlier while I was at work. He was in the intensive care unit.

Over the phone, David's speech was labored. His nurses had him hooked to a machine that allowed him to breathe easier. A few times during our conversation, he had to pause to take a deep breath. He told me he was recovering from a surgery. His doctors had snipped off a small part of his liver. A few weeks before, his oncologist had ordered a full-body PET scan. David was nervous about the meeting to discuss the results. Called it "his day of reckoning." He promised he would call me to share the results regardless of if they were good or bad. But he didn't call. Days passed. Then a week. I didn't call because I figured he received some awful news and was shutting himself off to cope. I knew how that felt, so I wanted to respect his need for space. Eventually, I gutted it up and called him. Davidcito told me the bad news: his anal cancer had spread to his liver.

When he rang me from his ICU room, David told me the procedure was a success. The surgeons had removed the cancerous part of his liver and sewn him up without incident. But the following day, while recuperating in his hospital room, David's heart rate spiked. This prompted his move to the ICU. He asked if I could visit him soon. I was worried that this might be it for him. I asked if I could visit him later that day, after my early-evening therapy session.

Once I walked through the hospital's sliding doors, I turned to the left, then to the right. David told me the ICU was on the fourth floor, but in what wing? Being on the other side—a visitor instead of a patient—was a little confusing. Up until that day, I was somewhat unaware that there *even was* another hospital wing, since my sole purpose in visiting Mt. Zion was to receive my radiation treatments in their basement. I walked to the elevators to the left—the wing I was accustomed to migrating to. The elevator doors opened to the reception area for the oncology department. *Whoops.* I doubled back and walked to the other wing. The elevator doors opened to a quiet, blue-green hallway that was good at producing echoing footsteps. I followed the signs to the intensive care unit.

The thick metallic doors into the ward were shut. I placed my hands on the cold door to peek through its window. It seemed like the right place: the rows of rooms were cordoned off with transparent vinyl curtains. The ward seemed still and serious, like a morgue or a place where people were kept during a contagion outbreak. A sign advised all visitors to have clean hands before entering. No sick visitors were allowed. Another sign by the doors directed visitors to call a nurse inside the unit to receive entrance. I lifted the phone nearby and dialed the unit. All that procedure, all that security, all that precaution frightened me. My friend must be in bad shape if he was taken here, I thought. I took a deep breath while the phone rang. I was afraid of what I might find inside.

A woman answered and allowed me in. The automated doors slowly opened as if I had incanted the correct spell. A nurse met me by the entrance. "David will be pleased to have a visitor," she said with a bright smile that further weirded me out. I felt like I had been swept into a dream that had the chilling pretense of a nightmare.

Parting the vinyl curtain, she escorted me into David's room. He lay in a bed inclined at a sixty-degree angle. David wore his trademark round black glasses that I could pick out in a crowd. An elevated hospital tray was at his reach. A spirometer and a small carton of orange juice with a straw rested on it. He was aglow from the pale sunlight that seeped through a long window, which I immediately noted faced west, looking out over Divisadero Street. He was staring into the waning light. Plastic tubes were inserted into his nostrils. They were connected to an oxygen tank. A few machines stood beside his bed. One continuously beeped, measuring his heart rate.

"Juan!" David said, turning to me. His voice was weak and diminished.

"Hi, David." I took a tentative step to his side once I saw that he expected a hug. I wasn't sure if I could touch him.

I carefully leaned over to embrace him. He had to struggle to put his arms around me. The hug we shared was not like the ones we gave each other in the men's locker room, or the hugs we had when we met for breakfast back in mid-February.

"My, you look dapper," he said when I stood back beside the serving tray at the foot of his bed. With my hands tucked into my coat pockets, I gave an "oh, you" titter.

"Had to go to work and earn some peanuts!" I said, rocking on my loafer heels. Despite the unfamiliar setting and the bleak circumstances behind my visit, I felt sprightly, as if I were some good boy gunning for Employee of the Month. "I brought some gifts for you!"

David mustered some excitement as I set my shoulder bag on the tray. I reached in and handed him Yiyun Li's *A Thousand Years of Good Prayers* along with two fine milk-chocolate bars I bought after my therapy session.

"I haven't read that book, but I've heard good things about it," I said.

"Oh, thank you, Juan," he said, turning his gaze to the chocolate bars, "but I can't eat those. They're gonna have me on a boring diet for at least a month."

I had already figured that he would not be able to eat solids. Around that time, I had proposed a "More Chocolates, Less Beer" campaign for myself in therapy with Akhila. I figured some chocolate could be good for David, too.

"You should keep them," I said. "You can look forward to gobbling them someday soon."

David smiled.

"Thank you for the gifts, for visiting."

"How are you feeling?" I asked, still feeling unusually giddy.

"Ah, guy," he said, shaking his head, holding his hands out. "The surgery, which lasted *four and a half hours*, went well. The pain isn't so bad because they got me hooked on morphine."

"Ooh, morphine," I said, turning my head and mischievously raising a brow. Right after I said that, I regretted it. David had a dark, witty, sardonic sense of humor like me, but I was fearful I had gone too far in joking about his present predicament, which was *not* funny whatsoever. Thankfully, he chortled and rolled with it.

Then, David trailed off and told me he had become obsessed with American frontiersmen. The myth of the Old West, the promised land it was purported to be. His ancestors were among those immigrants, after all. There was a sense of awe and defeat in his voice when he talked about all the dreams those early European immigrants had about California. While he spoke, I just nodded and listened, but it troubled me that David had become fixated on *that* topic; I could not help but think about the symbolism of the West: the fading sun over the Pacific, the twilight before complete dark. I did not want my friend to think about his dashed dreams of good health. I did not want him to think about death as though it was around the corner. I did not want him to give up, though I felt that he wanted to. I could hear it in his weary voice.

Before long, David told me about the hallucinations the morphine was causing. His eyes widened as he stared at the smoke detector on the wall in front of him. He told me its blinking red light was messing with him at night, that he had heard roars and trumpets coming from it. Having done his share of hallucinogens in his life, David knew they were not real. But nevertheless, it frightened him. I gave a sympathetic murmur as I listened, but the further his ramble went, the more I wanted to bound out of there. What unhinged me the most was the terror in his eyes, how large they bulged when he looked up at the smoke detector. "Maybe the nurses can cover it?" I asked. "That might not be a bad idea," he said.

David continued on, again bringing up how the surgery had lasted four and a half hours. "I really hope it works, baby, because I just can't go through another surgery like this again."

Then the beeping on his machine flatlined. It made a droning sound as if he was dead. Though I was startled, I didn't flip out only because David paid no attention to it. The nurse power walked in, all chipper yet commanding. She pressed a few buttons on the machine.

"We need to hook you back up to the oxygen machine because your heart rate just shot up," she said, handling the tubes and wires by the oxygen tank.

"Oh—I couldn't tell," David said with nonchalance.

The nurse told me our visit had to come to an end.

"David," the nurse said, "you *have* to keep doing your breathing exercises so we can get you off that machine and out of here." He nodded with an "I know, I know" expression. I gave David a hug good-bye, then left.

As I walked down the dimly lit blue-green hallway, I stared at the floor. I was trying to determine how I should feel. *Could this be the last time I will see him alive? No . . . No.* It just didn't *feel* like it would be. It was a completely intuitive feeling, though I was concerned his heart could give out if it continued to wildly fluctuate.

When I stepped into the elevator, I felt a sense of satisfaction come over me. I was pleased I had shown David I would be there for him.

But then I remembered those eyes of his. Desperate. Reaching. Frantic.

I had never seen a gaze like that.

The Big, Big Fear

AROUND THE TIME I visited David in the hospital, I finally had a dream starring Mr. Hodgkins. In the dream, it was nighttime. I was walking in a cold, dimly lit room that resembled a commercial kitchen. Bluish moonlight seeped through a skylight. A long, silver table gleaming with a spectral luminescence stood between me and Mr. Hodgkins. He slowly paced along the other side of the table, a few feet ahead of me. The clacking sound of his shoes echoed through the room. I stepped up my pace, glaring at him. Mr. Hodgkins looked much different from the version of him I had created. He was much taller—at least a foot taller than me. Gone was his trademark derby hat. Instead, his full set of jet-black hair was slicked back. He wore a black, Draculaesque robe. When I caught up, adjacent to him, I could see half of his face alit in moonlight. He looked pale, ancient, weathered, his eyes thin, piercing slits with a yellow, catlike glow. It was a devil version of Mr. Hodgkins— all-knowing, immortal. Despite this, when we neared the end of the metallic table, I shoved it aside, clanging against the tiles, so I could pounce on him.

That's when I awoke beside Paola in her bed, facing her, my hands shoving her like I had pushed that table in my dream. I gasped. My eyes were wide open as she also startled awake in the morning dark.

"You had a nightmare!" she said.

"Yeah, I just had a nightmare of Mr. Hodgkins," I said, turning away. "But he was basically the devil."

The pounding in my chest lessened as I lay on my side. I replayed the dream—his face, his archetypal appearance—before I went back to sleep.

✖

Shortly after I had this nightmare, I tried out sandplay therapy with Akhila. In her study, we stood around a large sandtray. Beside it was a bin teeming with toys and figurines. She told me to grab the toys that I was drawn to. I was smiley as I forked through the bin and recognized a few figurines. "Oh, Macho Man!" I said before I grabbed the muscled figurine of the famous wrestler.

These were the other toys I picked out to create my scene:

• Thumper the rabbit
• a rosy-cheeked clown
• a one-and-a-half-foot-long snake
• a gramophone
• an evil gremlin-like doll
• two black-winged devils

I placed the sprightly Thumper near the middle of the sandtray. Macho Man and the clown flanked the rabbit, who stared up with adorable eyes, one big paw lifted and ready to thump the ground. Behind them lay the snake, which I placed belly-up. Thumper and his friends faced the imposing gremlin-like doll and his two winged devils. A gramophone stood to the side, facing all of them.

Crossing my arms proudly, I explained to Akhila that Thumper was me. The snake signified the bad habits and destructive thoughts I was trying to shed myself of. Macho Man stood for my tough side; the cheerful clown symbolized the eight-year-old self I wanted to tap into more often. They were "my crew." The gremlin-like doll was Mr. Hodgkins and the devils his obedient minions.

"That's interesting that your crew is facing Mr. Hodgkins and his minions instead of having them behind you," Akhila said, standing beside me.

"Hmmm," I said with a downward glance. "Well, I guess I did that because I presume—at some point—that I'll have to go through that again. That I'll relapse."

Cosmic Fairy Dust

ONE NIGHT, I stayed up late in my bedroom, putzing around on my laptop. While I browsed through my pictures, I came across the ones my mom took of me during my eleventh infusion. I brought this up in therapy a few days later.

"She took seven pictures," I told Akhila, who looked grim as she faced me, sitting on her couch. "I'm passed out in four of them, my head slumped to the side, an IV pricked in my arm. And I look so help-less. So . . . vulnerable." I stared off toward the window behind Akhila. My eyes were welling up with tears. "And it just felt so unreal to look at them, thinking that *that really* happened to me," I said, crying. "And there's *nothing* I can do about that."

During that therapy session, I came to realize that the main reason I was there with Akhila was because I didn't want to feel sad about that period of my life. I was there so she could help me build an armor for postcancer life (i.e., the rest of my life). Much like the late writer Kath-erine Russell Rich, who wrote, "Happiness is my protection, my talis-man," in her fantastic memoir *The Red Devil: To Hell with Cancer—and Back*, I felt like my happiness and contentment was the strongest tonic against getting another life-threatening malady. By then I had encoun-tered a common cancer survivor pitfall: freaking the fuck out for prac-tically *any* bodily misfire. After a night out with my coworkers during which I did a shot of tequila and took a few drags from a cigarette (though I knew it was unwise to smoke a cigarette, I took a few drags because I still felt this stupid compulsion to demonstrate to myself that I was physically unaltered from my battle against lymphoma), I awoke the next morning with tightness near where my tumor had been. *Oh my god, oh my god, oh my god, oh my god—the cancer's back*, I thought. The return of Mr. Hodgkins, like a corporeal terminator emerging from the pile of rubble of his bombed-out cavern. This fear—of getting cancer again—has never left.

With Akhila, I brought up the deliriously glorious month of March when I was told I was lymphoma-free. That mesospheric high I felt on life had long since faded. I knew that such a zenith of happiness would be an anomaly in my life, like a comet seen once or twice in a lifetime. Evan Handler recounted a similar reaction in his memoir once he first entered remission. I knew myself well enough to know that I would likely feel the same, unable to grasp that whirlwind of giddiness for long. Life can never be that good for that long—not when everything is in a state of impermanence. All I had left from that time was the memory of being resplendently happy to be alive and healthy. I told Akhila that if I was truly smart, I would conceive a way to keep the "cosmic fairy dust" of that comet alive and present throughout the rest of my life, as if I were watching it shoot off into the nebulae through a telescope.

And that *has* been the challenge in postcancer life—how to assemble that telescope, remembering to peer through it periodically. Drinking less, exercising more, eating healthier, and consuming foods and supplements with anticancerous properties have been simple changes to implement with time. (I still ride my bicycle a lot and try to hit the gym at least twice a week. And I mostly stick to beer so it's easier to know when to cut myself off. In fact, nowadays, I almost always cough nervously just before I leave home to go out drinking with a friend. When I was young, I used to relish losing control while I was drunk. Now it scares me.) But learning to be happy with myself and grateful for what I have will always be a challenge.

Low Sperm Count Blues

DURING THE SUMMER of 2010, I made an appointment with my doctor to get my sperm count tested. Two weeks later, my doctor called on a weekday morning. He caught me at home as I was leaving for work. He told me my sperm count was notably low, probably due to the chemotherapy I received. He told me that the average male has over twenty-two million sperm in an ejaculate; mine had one and a half million. Not much of a reproductive wallop. More like a wilting flower with that sad "whomp-whomp" trombone sound.

After we ended our call, I sat on my bed. I was wearing my black pea coat, fancy brown slacks, and oxfords. I stared off at the wall for minutes. Up until that point, I felt like I had come out of that battle for my life physically intact. At the gym, I had whipped myself into mightier shape than my precancer self. I was routinely cycling seven miles on the exercise bike in about twenty-one minutes with a respectable amount of resistance, then pounding out a mile and a half on the treadmill in less than thirteen minutes. It saddened me to know that a part of my body had probably become depleted due to lymphoma, that it was possible that my power to impregnate a woman had been wrenched from me.

Before I walked to the office, I stopped at the liquor store by the West Oakland BART station. I bought a pocket-sized bottle of Jameson to spike my morning coffee. Why the fuck not? I thought. I was well aware that drinking was a piss-poor, illusory means of coping with the sadness within me, but I felt the need to do something stupid. Something absurd. Why not when our world is fucking absurd? And after everything that had happened to me, what did it matter?

A month later, while having dinner with my parents at our home in Fremont, I told them I got my sperm count tested. By then, I had gotten over my low sperm count blues (which I think would be a great title for a lo-fi blues ditty à la Skip James). But they became long-faced—especially my mom—when I told them.

I have no regrets about choosing not to freeze my sperm. I would prefer to adopt. (It's turned out well for a few people I know.) And I would like to someday. It might be the most selfless, loving thing I could ever do.

Shout at the Devil!

FOR HALLOWEEN FESTIVITIES in the city, Paola invited me to meet up with her friends at the 500 Club for some drinks. It was one of my favorite bars in the city, a short walk from home.

Paola was dressed as a bumblebee with bouncy antennae and fairy wings. She stood by the bar with three of her friends. I stalked into the bar dressed as the Grim Reaper—a skeletal mask covering my face, a plastic scythe in hand. The black graduation robe I had shelled out a hundred bucks for was a superb garment for my deathmonger costume. To my surprise and delight, Paola didn't recognize me when I stepped over to her side. She became uneasy and looked over her shoulder at me with a who-the-fuck-is-this-guy face. When I said, "Hey Paola," she wrinkled her brow at me. Once I took off my mask, she gave a sigh of relief.

I put my mask back on after I ordered a pint of beer. Standing by the counter, I managed to drink it through the mouth opening of my mask. A guy standing next to me told me I looked freaky drinking with that mask on. I laughed and said, "Why thank you."

An hour later, inspired by a few pints, I borrowed Paola's fairy wings. I put them on and twirled and headbanged with scythe in hand while my jukebox selection, Mötley Crüe's "Shout at the Devil," boomed through the bar. Across the bar in the adjacent pool room, a group of blondes pointed and stared at me with fascinated horror. I laughed heartily while I raised my scythe into the air when Vince Neil screamed "Shout at the Devil!" I was so pleased with myself. In therapy, which I ceased after only five months, Akhila and I talked about how I should find healthy ways to express the darkness I would always have inside. She would have been proud. That Grim-Reaper-with-fairy-wings dance to "Shout at the Devil" was a fine example of how it could be done.

As the song finished playing, I roared and strummed on the scythe as if it were a mighty Gibson Les Paul guitar.

Despedida

BACK IN LATE September, David and I met up for lunch. I strolled over to the condominium he shared with his partner, Jimmy, a few blocks from my home. The sun shined brightly above while I waited for David outside the main lobby. I had not seen him since his surgery earlier that summer. His recovery was a bit rough; he had to stay in the hospital for a few weeks. Worse, the doctors found that his anal cancer had grown back. In an e-mail, David wrote, "This is a bummer, no pun, of the big deal kind. Any further radiation is out because I was over-radiated last time; chemo has a 30 percent chance of affecting the tumor." Once he received that news, David and Jimmy hit the road (made "a lot of car journeys, not good on my ass") to visit and reminisce with their friends.

I could feel my heart drop when I saw David trudge across the lobby, smiling at me. He seemed so frail compared to the time back in March when I met up with him and my friend Jonny to watch *The Red Shoes* at the Castro Theatre. Once he opened the lobby door, we shared a long embrace. Then I put my arm around him to help him descend the three steps from the entrance, all the while thinking, *Please don't fall, David, please don't fall*, because I was afraid he would hurt himself, and if he did I would turn into a sobbing, sobbing mess.

Together, we slowly walked out to the street.

"How ya doin' today?" I asked, staring at the pavement in front of us. "I bet you're tired of people asking you that, huh?"

David gave a laugh.

"Oh, baby, it's been a wild ride lately, but I'm feeling better today," he said.

While we walked up to the corner of 15th and Dolores, David told me more about the spread of his cancer. The tone of his voice was not somber or dejected when he told me how grim his prognosis was. Instead, his voice was simply matter-of-fact, which made it more difficult for me to take in. By the time we got to the crosswalk, my eyes were filling with tears I was trying hard to hold back, especially when he told me, "We all have to go sometime."

As we crossed the avenue, David hooked his arm around mine. I could feel myself lighten when he did. I looked back at a driver that stopped to allow us to cross. In that moment, I could see myself and David through his eyes. I felt so honored and fortunate to be able to care for this beautiful man who put his arm around mine.

"I used to think that cancer would never get me," he said. "Not David Hardy! I'm too tough. But—I found out that we're all *vulnerable*. All mortal."

"Mortals!" I said, shaking my fist.

Once we crossed the street, David said, "Well, let me just get this out of the way: things are not good. And so how are you?"

I knew he wanted a reprieve from himself, so I blabbed and blabbed about my life. I told him things were crazy on my end, as usual. (I felt self-conscious after I blurted this out because I knew it was not nearly as crazy as everything he must have been going through.) I told him it was especially nutty in the love department during the past three weeks. I told him I broke up with Paola the night before and needed to make this one stick. Since David seemed relieved to hear about someone else's life besides his own, I went on a tangent about my love life by bringing up the book I had been reading, Louis-Ferdinand Céline's *Journey to the End of the Night*.

"I put the book down because I thought it was boring, but it did have a few good lines," I said. "He had a line that said something like, 'Love is harder to let go of than life.' And I think he was pretty much right. At least to me."

David grimaced and shook his head.

"Mmm, I don't agree with that," he said. "Being in the position I'm in—losing my life—I can tell you that it's much harder to let go of than love."

I hung my head and murmured. I felt bad for being so oblivious, for bringing up the struggle he was going to lose.

We ate at Chilango's, a Mexican restaurant that had just opened in the Castro neighborhood. We were seated next to the windows. David-cito was excited about our meal. For weeks he had been put on a restrictive diet that was easier on his digestive system. He was determined to eat and drink whatever he damn well pleased, even though his butt would not be happy with him later. We both ordered a delicious plate of huevos rancheros. He drank a bottle of Bohemia, which I told him was my father's favorite beer. I had told David that he was only a few months older than my dad, who was also born in 1939.

While I sipped on my glass of sangria, David stared out the window at the people passing by.

"All this time, I could have started to look back over my life," he said, turning to look down at the table. "I should have done this, I wish I could have done that, or I wish I wouldn't have been so fucked up when I was with this person. But I don't have any regrets about how things turned out."

"Yeah, regret's the worst thing."

"That's true, but now I think that expectation—when you hope and hope and expect something to turn out a certain way but then it doesn't—is the worst thing. I think that's the one thing that has caused me the most pain in life."

It saddened me to hear this. I understood what he was talking about. We both looked downward.

"I've got some good news, David," I said with a soft voice, a faint smile.

"Well, I love to hear good news for you, my dear."

"I've been awarded an artist residency in Taos, New Mexico. It's for *thirteen weeks*." David raised his glass to congratulate me.

"You're gonna love it there. It's absolutely gorgeous, and there are some *real* hippies over there. Believe me—they will make you miss the normalcy of San Francisco."

I laughed.

Once we started talking about New Mexico and the Southwest, he brought up Sedona, Arizona. "The drive from Flagstaff to Sedona is the most beautiful I've ever seen," he told me while I sat with rapt attention. "Sedona is so beautiful you'll want to weep when you get there." I vowed to myself then that someday I would make that drive through the Monument Valley. Beholding that landscape would be my way of honoring David, the life I still carried within.

When we walked down Church Street back to his home, I felt an overwhelming sense of desperation that I had never quite felt in my life. It kind of felt like watching a World Cup elimination match in which your team is down by a goal, the seconds on the clock ticking away in the extra minutes, one eye on the ball, the other on the referee, dreading that he will raise his hand and blow the whistle to end the game. But this was no game. With David walking beside me, I kept thinking *this is it*—the last moments I will have with him. I should be documenting this. Photographing him. Capturing him before he's gone. I had taken one picture of him at the restaurant, but I also had my voice recorder in my pocket. I wanted to take more photos and record his voice, but I felt terrible about asking him, about possibly making him even sadder. So I refrained. (But I did go home and immediately jotted down notes and snippets of our conversation.)

During our walk, David told me I was the only person he had been able to tell that he was dying. He was able to because I was like a stranger, yet tied to him because of our mutual death-blooming-inside-my-body experience. When we approached the condominiums, he said, "Ah shit, I'm shitting myself." After I put my hand on his back as we crossed the street, he said, "You're the only one I tell these things." I smirked. I took it as a compliment. Other folks in my life had told me that they felt like they could discuss anything with me.

To my surprise, neither of us became a blubbering mess when we hugged good-bye at the front entrance. But when I turned to leave, I began to replay a few of the things he had just told me. Consumed in my thoughts, I walked down Guerrero Street, the street I marched on the night I was diagnosed with lymphoma. I remembered when he told me that broken hopes could be the worst thing. Halfway down the block, I ducked beneath a building. I buried my face in my hands and sobbed. I couldn't help but remember when I first met David, when we embraced in the locker room and he told me, "We're going to make it."

A month later, I came over to David and Jimmy's to have dinner with them. Although back in June he sounded reluctant to have another surgery, David agreed to undergo a procedure on November 2 to attempt to remove his malignant tumor. It was a final hope that did not bloom.

Months later, in April 2011, I began to come over to their condominium on weekdays to take David for a walk around the block. I was working two part-time gigs: an evening job proofreading translations of legal documents, and consulting for a small nonprofit in Oakland. Between them, I had an unusual schedule that allowed me to have a number of days off during the week. By then, David was in worse shape. His anal canal was in ruins. It was painful for him to sit. He couldn't go to the bathroom, either, so he had to have a urinary catheter and drain bag attached to him at all times, which an in-home nurse emptied every morning. His doctors could not guesstimate how much time he had left.

David and I would gingerly walk around the block, his arm nestled around mine. His gray hair was cropped. His beard had grown out. He would tell me about his siblings and nieces who were coming to visit from his home state of Utah. He told me about the ultraconservative, religious community he had fled decades before for the freedom he found in San Francisco. He would make me laugh with a few of his stories, especially some funny ones about all the good times he had with weed and mushrooms. (One of my favorite stories of his was the time he blared an opera from a furniture store he used to work for in Salt Lake City so he could march out to the middle of the street and move his hands as if he were conducting the music.) I remember how tranquil and peaceful our walks seemed. Birds chirping in the trees we passed. Sunlight trickling through the leaves. It felt nourishing to slow down with David.

After our strolls, I would sit and talk with David in his living room until he felt too fatigued. Sitting on a leather couch, I often held his warm hand while he sat beside me on a super-soft cushion. Sometimes he would sigh about his state and shake his head and tell me how hard it is to let go. I would squeeze his hand and meet his eyes.

I remember the last time we were together in his living room. David told me, "I've learned that there's nothing to be afraid of. Have no fear about *anything*. No fear." When he said this, he squeezed my hand and looked into my eyes, as if saying, "Don't ever forget this."

Two weeks later, on May 9, 2011, I called David from my bedroom. I had not heard from him in a week. Jimmy answered. I was startled to find him home on a Monday. I asked if I could speak to David. "Oh, I have some bad news. David passed away on Saturday night," he told me. I could feel the breath come out of me. I didn't know how to respond other than to say how unfortunate that was to hear. Jimmy told me how swiftly David deteriorated after his family left, how awful it all turned, how David could make little sense in the end. He told me David must have felt bad that he couldn't say good-bye to me. He knew how grateful David was to have me in his life at the end. Jimmy said there would be a memorial in a few weeks. I told him I wouldn't miss it for anything.

After we hung up, I looked out my window toward David and Jimmy's home. I sat on my lounge chair and stared at the sunlight falling into my room. No one else was home. I peered up to the cloudless sky above the dilapidated buildings behind our house. I cried. With my flip-flops on, I grabbed my iPod and walked out to the back patio. I played John Coltrane's "My Favorite Things" while I collected my white laundry from the washer outside.

While hanging my laundry on the clotheslines, a crow flew down between the buildings that surrounded our backyard. The crow perched on the metal fence that separated the neighboring backyard. It was no more than fifteen feet away from me, facing me at eye level. It remained there for a good twenty to thirty seconds, even after I cawed at it (which is something I like to do now with crows. I am no longer afraid of them. In fact, I love them. I love playfully cawing at them whenever I see one, in the silly hopes that they will caw back at me). The crow flew up and disappeared into the thicket of leaves from the small tree in the neighbor's yard. While I hung my socks to McCoy Tyner's piano solo, I peered over at the bird. Shortly after it flapped up into the tree, the crow flew off, above the roof of our house. For the briefest of seconds, a tiny brown sparrow swooped out from our roof to playfully chase and circle the crow before it settled on the edge of the roof of the dilapidated house behind ours. While I looked up at it, the black bird almost appeared to be peering down at me. Then it flew off. Seconds later, I saw it flying south, up above the backyards of the neighboring houses.

Besides the timing, what made this visit most unusual is that I had never seen a crow descend to our patio. Our backyard—as well as the two neighboring ones—was a popular urban cove for pigeons. Like an oasis from the city's bustle. From my bedroom, I saw and heard pigeons all the time during the year I lived in that house. They cooed to one another, flapped from roof to roof, or strutted about in a mating dance on the building behind us. On occasion, doves and English sparrows joined them, but that was the only time any bird remained that close to me in our back patio. Crows were no strangers to the neighborhood. On a few occasions, I saw a murder of crows perched on the wires that crisscrossed the houses on our block of Lexington Street. But I never saw another crow in our back patio again.

Flabbergasted, my jaw hanging, eyes fluttering, I walked back to my room to text three of my most trusted friends. I told them what had just happened. I didn't know what that crow's visit meant—if it meant anything. My friends Scott, Tagi, and Carlisle—an atheist, spiritual but not religious, and agnostic—all wrote to say that it seemed like my friend David had come back to say good-bye. It warmed me to read this because that is what I felt in my heart, what I wanted to believe.

Once I put my phone down, I looked past the sunlight streaming through the window. I was searching for the crow. *Come back*, I was thinking. *Come back*. It never did.

And so, my friend David was gone.

But I am still here.

Acknowledgments

FIRST AND FOREMOST, I want to thank my parents. None of this would have been possible without all your love and support. Les quiero con todo mi corazón. Un abrazote for my sisters and greater family for all your support and for always allowing me to be the wacky one.

To all the nurses, doctors, and medical-care providers who tended to me, I am forever humbled by your kindness, your devotion, and the sacrifice you make in caring for others. I live to honor all the care you gave to me.

To my writing community, a big shout-out to my VONA family, especially Tara Dorabji, Nayomi Munaweera, Rita Chang, Lisa D. Gray, the Sunday Stories Writing Group, and my VONA '09 Memoir Workshop class. Much love to my homeboy (and savior from lumber-necked, leather-clad, urban behemoths!) Scott Russell Duncan for his bountiful generosity and camaraderie. A big thank you to my homies Justin "J-Oro" Goldman and Eric Taylor Aragón for their feedback and friendship. Much love and gratitude to my Saint Mary's community: my wonderful mentors Marilyn Abildskov and Wesley Gibson, and the mighty Pen Ultimate Longs: Rosa del Duca, Erin McCabe, and Risa Nye. I also want to thank Jane Vandenburgh and Leslie Carol Roberts. A big shout-out to the Nonfictionistas, especially Xochitl Magaly Perales: I am forever indebted for your kindness, compassion, and support after I was given my bad news.

I also want to acknowledge and thank Deborah Raye Jackson and, most especially, Lezly Hawkins for opening my world to so many wonderful books and films, which was instrumental in my development as a reader and writer. Thank you to Stephen Gutierrez for being the first person to encourage me to continue writing. I also wanna give a shout-out to Tagi Qolouvaki, Cynthia Polutanovich, Amber Lamprecht, and Kelly Gleason for their friendship and support during a difficult period in my life. (And thank you for your persistence in trying to break my propensity for adverbs, Kelly!)

Thank you to Michael Knight and the Helene Wurlitzer Foundation of New Mexico for giving me invaluable time and space to write and heal. And thank you to Nicholas Bocek and my Proofington homies for supporting my artistic endeavors. A big, big thank you to Ethan Ly.

I want to thank my fantastic editor Elise McHugh (you're a peach and a half!) and the team at the University of New Mexico Press. I am so grateful for all of your work.

David Hardy—you will always be remembered.

And finally, I want to give my unending gratitude to my sweetheart, Maria Bustamante. I love who I am when I'm with you, and this book would not have been possible without your love.